It's time to explode

If you think that menopause necessarily means suffering from symptoms such as hot flashes, vaginal dryness, depression, and irritability, think again...
Hormone additive therapy (also known as hormone replacement therapy) offers many menopausal women much-needed relief from these and other bothersome symptoms, while many other women going through menopause never suffer discomfort in the first place.

If you think that *all* menopausal women need hormone therapy, think again...
It's perfectly *normal* for postmenopausal women to have lower levels of estrogen. In fact, the majority of menopausal women do perfectly well without hormone therapy, provided they enter menopause in optimal health and maintain good health throughout their menopausal years.

If you think you don't need hormone additive therapy because you don't have any of the classic symptoms of menopause, think again...
Heart disease and osteoporosis are the silent, long-term complications of menopause. If you are at high risk for either of these conditions, you may want to consider taking hormones.

The question is, should *you* be treated, and how?

ESTROGEN: YES OR NO?

(Published simultaneously with the authors' comprehensive guidebook, *Menopause and Midlife Health*)

Illustrations by Aher/Donnell Studios

Chart graphics by Douglas Reinke

Morris Notelovitz, M.D., Ph.D. and Diana Tonnessen

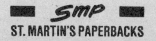

SMP

ST. MARTIN'S PAPERBACKS

Many of the designations used by manufacturers and sellers to distinguish their products are claimed as trademarks or registered trademarks. Where those designations appear in this book and the authors were aware of a trademark claim, the designations have been printed in initial capital letter (e.g., Anaprox).

Estrogen: Yes or No? is adapted from the authors' comprehensive guidebook, *Menopause and Midlife Health*, copyright © 1993 and published by St. Martin's Press.

ESTROGEN: YES OR NO?

ISBN: 0-312-95105-1

Printed in the United States of America

St. Martin's Paperbacks edition/May 1993

10 9 8 7 6 5 4 3 2

Note to the reader:

It is advisable for the reader to seek the guidance of a licensed physician or gynecologist before implementing any of the programs or techniques described in this book. Needless to say, prescription drugs should be used only on the advice of a licensed physician. Do *not* make any changes in your medication regimen without consulting your doctor, and contact your physician promptly if you have any reason to suspect that you suffer from one or more of the diseases or health problems described in the book. Neither this nor any other book should be used as a substitute for professional medical care or treatment.

Contents

Preface

When in 1989 we started writing our book *Menopause and Midlife Health* (St. Martin's Press, 1993), we were advised not to use the word *menopause* in the title because it would be a turnoff to readers. Menopause was simply not a subject open for discussion—even as little as a few years ago. Yet we knew from our experience with more than 11,000 women at our clinic (the Women's Medical and Diagnostic Center and Climacteric Clinic in Gainesville, Florida—the first clinic in the country to cater exclusively to women in midlife) that there was a hunger and a great need for information about menopause and about the most widely prescribed treatment for menopausal symptoms: estrogen.

Since that time, the media and masses of baby boomers entering the menopausal years have helped to make the "M" word a household word. Two times in as many years, menopause was featured on the cover of *Newsweek* magazine. It's been discussed on television talk shows and has made headlines in newspapers and on national network news. Then in 1992, journalist Gail Sheehy broke the silence—and sales records—with her book *The Silent Passage: Menopause*, a best-selling book with "menopause" in the title. At last, it has become safe—even socially acceptable—to talk about menopause, one of the most important biological milestones of a woman's life.

What hasn't changed is the need for good, solid, scientifically based information about menopause, which is why we wrote *Menopause and Midlife Health*, the most comprehensive guide to date on menopause and on keeping healthy in your middle and later years. The concept of that book—that you *can* prepare for a comfortable menopause and enjoy good health in your later years, what we call "climacteric medicine"—is based on more than twenty years of research involving thousands of women at our clinic. Established in 1986, the Women's Medical and Diagnostic Center was (as we mentioned earlier) the first clinic in the country devoted entirely to meeting the health needs of women in the middle years, from ages thirty-five to sixty-five. The Climacteric Clinic is the research arm of the Center, where ongoing studies are furthering our knowledge about menopause and its effects on a woman's health.

When in 1992 Premarin (a form of estrogen commonly used to treat menopausal symptoms) became the most widely prescribed drug in the United States, we recognized another need: the need for women in the middle years to have objective, unbiased, up-to-date information about postmenopausal estrogen, information they need to make an intelligent decision about whether or not to take postmenopausal estrogen. This is a question that virtually every woman will have to face at some time in her life. So we have pulled together the most relevant information from *Menopause and Midlife Health* and are presenting it in this smaller handbook for those of you who must answer the more immediate question of whether or not to start postmenopausal estrogen therapy.

As you will learn in the pages to come, estrogen is just one of many options available to help make your menopause more manageable and to prevent its two most serious long-term health risks—heart disease and osteoporosis. We hope this book whets your appetite for more information, and recommend that you refer to *Menopause and Midlife Health*, where you'll find our complete program for good health in your middle and later years, and for making these years the prime years of your life.

Introduction

You have probably heard about some of the wonderful things postmenopausal hormone therapy can do for you: Estrogen relieves hot flashes. Estrogen can keep you looking and *feeling* more youthful. Estrogen can revitalize your sex life. Is it all true?

Undoubtedly, you have also heard or read about some of the risks associated with hormone therapy. You're probably wondering: Does it cause heart attacks? What about the risk of cancer? Doesn't hormone therapy cause blood clots?

Estrogen: A Look Back

Much of the confusion surrounding estrogen arises from its checkered past. The last time estrogen enjoyed such widespread popularity was after the publication in 1963 of the book *Feminine Forever* (M. Evans & Co., Inc., New York) by Robert A. Wilson, M.D. In those days, estrogen was touted as a veritable fountain of youth, a wonder drug that could keep women looking and feeling "feminine forever." In fact, Wilson warned women that if they *didn't* take estrogen, they risked hopelessly withering into old age.

Then came reports in the late 1970s that estrogen, when taken alone by postmenopausal women who hadn't had a hysterectomy (surgical removal of the uterus), could cause endometrial cancer. Sales of estrogen plummeted as a wave of fear spread over women taking or thinking about taking this so-called wonder drug. Skepticism about estrogen grew when experts debated whether the "natural" estrogens prescribed for postmenopausal women might share some of the same long-term complications (an increased risk of blood clots, heart attacks, and strokes) associated with the early birth control pills, which contained high doses of synthetic estrogen and progestogen. Then came a highly publicized report in the late 1980s that estrogen might raise a postmenopausal woman's risk of breast cancer.

It's no wonder so many women today come to our clinic confused, scared, and armed with a healthy dose of skepticism about estrogen.

The Facts about Estrogen

Scientists and physicians have learned a lot about estrogen in the last twenty years. We now know that postmenopausal hormone therapy is an excellent way to relieve many of the discomforts of menopause, such as hot flashes and vaginal dryness. It's one of the most effective ways of slowing or stopping the loss of bone mass after menopause. There's mounting evidence that taking estrogen after menopause *prolongs* the apparent built-in protection against heart disease that premenopausal women enjoy. And yes, estrogen can keep your skin supple and younger looking (although it is *not* a cosmetic and we don't recommend that you use it in this way). As for the potential risks, when a progestogen is given along with estrogen to women with an intact uterus, the combination actually *protects* against endometrial cancer. Most studies today have shown that postmenopausal estrogen preparations don't substantially raise your risk of breast cancer, either. In effect, *estrogen as it is prescribed today is safer than ever before.*

But is estrogen the right treatment for *you*?

Replacing Hormones or Adding Them?

Before we help you answer that question, let's first clear up some confusion about the term most often used to describe postmenopausal hormones: *hormone replacement therapy*. Actually, this term is somewhat misleading because it suggests that you are replacing hormones that *should* be there. Technically, however, you're not replacing hormones; you're *adding* them. As you'll learn in the pages to come, the principal type of estrogen produced by your body changes after menopause. Postmenopausal women produce more *estrone* than *estradiol*, the predominant estrogen in premenopausal women. So if you were *replacing* hormones, you would actually receive more estrone than estradiol. However, most postmenopausal hormone therapy is intended to increase the blood levels of *estradiol*, the more potent of the two hormones.

The hormone progesterone is not normally produced at all in postmenopausal women. When progesterone is given to menopausal women (mainly for women with an intact uterus, and primarily to protect the lining of the uterus, the *endometrium*) synthetic types are prescribed.

While it may seem we're overly concerned with semantics, the issue runs far deeper than mere words. In a sense, the term *hormone replacement therapy* has become symbolic of a mind-set that has led to the medicalization of menopause. *Hormone replacement therapy* suggests that menopause is an illness that should be treated by replacing missing hormones, in the same way that diabetes is treated by replacing insulin. This has led to the belief—by some experts, at least—that *all* menopausal women should take hormones.

However, it's perfectly *normal* for postmenopausal women to have lower levels of estrogen. Most otherwise-healthy menopausal women don't experience any serious complications relating to the drop in estrogens after menopause. Indeed, the majority of menopausal women do perfectly well without hormone therapy *provided they enter menopause in optimal health and maintain good health throughout their postmenopausal years.*

For these reasons, we suggest you use the term *hormone additive therapy* (HAT) or *estrogen additive therapy* (EAT). Essentially, when physicians prescribe postmenopausal hormones, they are treating patients with drugs. There's nothing wrong with this so long as the benefits of the drug outweigh the risks.

Estrogen: Yes or No?

The question is, who should be treated, and how? Basically, four groups of women should consider treatment:

1. Women with symptoms of menopause, including
•hot flashes

●estrogen-related psychological symptoms, such as depression, irritability, confusion, mood swings, insomnia, and early morning awakenings

●vaginal dryness

●urinary tract symptoms that are *not* caused by a bacterial infection (what is known as *urethral syndrome*)

2. Women who experience an early menopause (either a "surgical" or natural menopause before age forty)

3. Women at risk of developing osteoporosis

4. Women at risk of cardiovascular disease

Of course, if you don't fall into one of these categories but wish to take hormone additive therapy, there's no reason not to (unless you're one of a minority of women for whom hormones are contraindicated). Neither is there hard evidence that by taking hormones, you'll be healthier or better off or will live longer than women who don't take hormones but adopt a healthy life-style in their middle and later years.

You can make a more informed decision by learning about the benefits and risks of hormone therapy, as well as alternatives available to you, all of which are described in the following chapters. If you do decide to take estrogen, you'll also learn about the various hormonal preparations available to you, whether you need to take a progestogen along with estrogen, what androgens can do for you, why and how you should be monitored by your doctor, and how to manage any possible side effects.

Should *you* take estrogen? Let us help you make the right choice.

CHAPTER 1

❈

What is Menopause?

There's really nothing mythical about menopause. It's simply a biological milestone marking the end of your reproductive years—just as your *menarche* (start of menstruation) marked the beginning.

Technically, your menopause lasts about a week—the week of your last menstrual period. But menopause is actually a culmination of changes in your ovaries that begin as early as your mid- to late thirties. Changes continue for up to fifteen years after menopause. This time in your reproductive life is known in medical circles as the *climacteric*. The entire spectrum of changes can be broken down into three stages: *premenopausal* (ages thirty to forty-five), *perimenopausal* (ages forty-five to fifty-five), and *postmenopausal* (ages fifty-five and older).

To understand what happens during your menopause, and the role of hormone additive therapy in your postmenopausal years, it first helps to know a little something about your reproductive system and menstrual cycle.

Your Reproductive System

Your reproductive system—ovaries, Fallopian tubes, uterus, and vagina, (see Figure 1-1)—begins to form

1

FIGURE 1-1. The Female Reproductive System

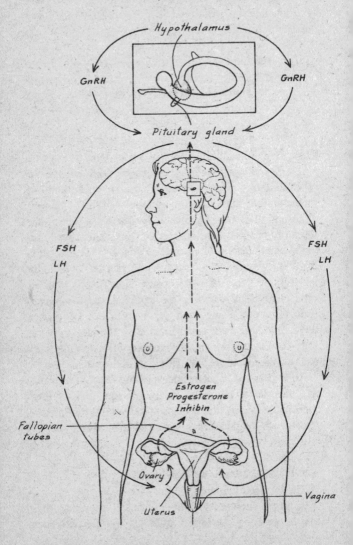

just seven or eight weeks after conception. By the time you are a seven-month-old fetus, your developing ovaries contain some 6 to 7 million eggs—a lifetime supply.

Throughout your life, the number of eggs diminishes, as they fail to develop and are reabsorbed back into the ovaries. By the time you are born, the number of eggs in your ovaries had already been reduced to about 2 million. When you reach puberty, your ovaries contain just 300,000 eggs, each surrounded by a casing of cells called a *follicle*.

During your childbearing years, only about 450 eggs will reach maturity and travel through the Fallopian tubes, where they can be fertilized by sperm. The rest slowly disintegrate. By the time you reach menopause, only about 3,000 ova remain.

How Your Reproductive Hormones Affect Your Menstrual Cycles

Your reproductive cycles are governed by hormones, chemical messengers that circulate throughout your bloodstream. Menstruation is initially triggered by hormones released from the *hypothalamus* years before you begin menstruating. The hypothalamus is the part of the brain that controls the endocrine (glandular) system and other bodily functions. Around the time of puberty, the hypothalamus begins releasing *gonadotropin-releasing hormone* (GnRH). Eventually, the hypothalamus produces enough GnRH to signal the pituitary gland to churn out *follicle-stimulating hormone* (FSH) and *luteinizing hormone* (LH). These two hormones communicate with your ovaries and help orchestrate your menstrual cycles.

In the first phase of your menstrual cycle, the *follicular phase*, your pituitary releases more FSH than LH. When FSH reaches your ovaries, it stimulates several eggs in the ovaries to grow and mature. The follicles surrounding the eggs absorb fluid and swell as they work their way to the surface of the ovary. Only one egg will grow sufficiently to ripen and be released from one of your ovaries. The others will slowly disintegrate.

As the follicles mature, they begin producing two types of *estrogen*: *estradiol* and *estrone*. These are very powerful hormones that stimulate the growth of specific cells in your body. Rising estrogen levels around the time of menarche (primarily estradiol) are responsible for the growth and maturation of your reproductive organs and your breasts. Estrogen also causes you to start storing fat in your buttocks and thighs. Estrogen stimulates bone growth and is largely responsible for the growth spurt associated with puberty. During each menstrual cycle, estrogen stimulates the cells lining your uterus (the *endometrium*) to grow and thicken, helping to prepare the uterus for pregnancy.

In the middle of your menstrual cycle, a surge of luteinizing hormone is released from the pituitary gland. It's not certain what signals the pituitary to suddenly secrete large amounts of LH, although it is suspected that rising levels of estrogen in the first phase of the cycle play a role. At any rate, the surge of LH causes rapid swelling of the follicle. It also causes the wall of the follicle to weaken. Eventually, the follicle ruptures and the ovum is released into your abdominal cavity—this is what is known as *ovulation*. The tiny hairs (or *cilia*) at the openings of the Fallopian tubes almost always draw the egg into the tube, where it can be fertilized.

In the second, or *luteal* phase of the menstrual cycle, the cells lining the space once occupied by the egg form the *corpus luteum*. Beginning just a few hours after ovulation, this mass of yellow cells secretes small amounts of estrogen and large amounts of progesterone, which further help thicken the uterine lining. The corpus luteum also produces *inhibin*. This hormone, along with estrogen and progesterone, signals the pituitary to stop secreting FSH and LH. As a result, both FSH and LH in the blood fall to very low levels.

The corpus luteum depends on FSH and LH to sustain it, and the low levels of FSH and LH cause the corpus luteum to degenerate. When this happens—about two days before menstruation—estrogen, progesterone, and inhibin levels fall. The sudden drop in estrogen and progesterone in turn, causes the endometrial lining to degenerate. A day or two later, the uterine lining is shed from the walls of the uterus, and you begin menstruating.

In the meantime, the pituitary gland, without estrogen, progesterone, and inhibin to suppress it, once again starts to secrete FSH and LH, stimulating more follicles and beginning the cycle all over again. The whole process takes about twenty-eight days. But a "normal" cycle can range from twenty-one to thirty-five days or more.

The Effects of Menopause on Your Reproductive Hormones

By your mid- to late thirties, the number of follicles in your ovaries has gradually declined. At about the same time, the remaining follicles become less responsive to FSH and LH. As a result of these changes, your ovaries produce less and less of the reproductive hormones estrogen and progesterone. A typical pattern: levels of estradiol begin to fall first, resulting in a gradual shortening of the luteal (second) phase of the menstrual cycle. This is followed by a drop in progesterone, which increases the overall length of the cycle and often results in heavier periods. In response to these changes, the pituitary secretes higher levels of FSH and LH to stimulate the ovaries.

You may not notice any difference in your menstrual cycles at first. But anywhere from two to eight years before menopause, your menstrual flow may change, becoming heavier one month and lighter the next. Your menstrual cycles themselves may become more erratic. You may even skip periods altogether.

Eventually (around age fifty-one for the average American woman), the levels of estrogen and progesterone produced by the ovaries drop so low that you stop menstruating altogether. You and your physician will know you've experienced menopause when you start having menopausal symptoms, such as hot flashes, or when you haven't had a period for twelve or more consecutive months. A blood test showing elevated FSH levels can also help your physician determine whether you are menopausal.

Although it may seem that your ovaries have completely shut down after menopause, our 1982 study of 145 pre- and postmenopausal women, supported by a grant from the National Institute on Aging, demonstrated that the ovaries still produce small amounts of estrogen (see Table 1-1). What's more, your ovaries continue to produce substantial amounts of the "male" androgens *testosterone* and *androstenedione* after menopause. Some of these hormones are converted to estrogen by body fat. In fact, most of the estrogen circulating in your bloodstream after menopause comes from these androgens. Your adrenal glands also produce minute amounts of estrogen.

TABLE 1-1. Pre- and Postmenopausal Hormone Levels

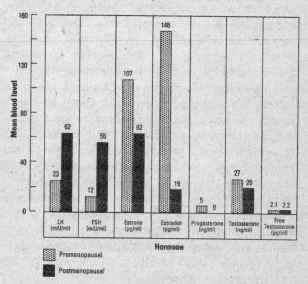

The predominant type of estrogen changes after menopause, too. Premenopausal women have higher levels of estradiol—the more potent of the two types of estrogen produced by the ovaries. After menopause, estrone is the principal type of estrogen circulating in your bloodstream.

On the other hand, since you've stopped ovulating

and no corpus luteum is formed, your ovaries produce virtually no progesterone or inhibin.

The Effect of Hormones on Your Heart and Bones

As you've already seen, the chief role of estrogen and progesterone is to help regulate your menstrual cycle and prepare your uterus for pregnancy. But like all hormones, these chemical messengers circulate throughout your body, interacting with other hormones and tissues, and with your body's metabolism. Estrogen *receptors*— specialized parts of cells that allow various hormones to lock into the cell and influence its activity—have been found in numerous tissues throughout the body, including your mucous membranes, your bladder, your breasts, your bones, your skin, and even the lungs and coronary arteries, which supply the heart muscle with nutrients and oxygen. This is why, when estrogen levels fall around the time of menopause, you may experience a number of physical (and sometimes psychological) changes. Some are nuisance symptoms, such as hot flashes and vaginal dryness, that let you know you're close to or just past menopause. Others are "silent" changes—and more serious.

Heart Disease

Postmenopausal women are more than twice as likely to develop heart disease as premenopausal women. This fact leads us to suspect that women are somehow protected against heart disease before menopause and that they lose this protection in the postmenopausal years.

We're still not sure why your risk of heart disease

rises after menopause. We do know, however, that estrogen affects blood cholesterol levels, a major risk factor for cardiovascular disease. Our 1982 study funded by the National Institute on Aging and other studies have found that total cholesterol levels of postmenopausal women are about 25 mg/dl higher than those of premenopausal women (see Table 1-2). And total cholesterol levels fall between 10 and 18 percent among postmenopausal women who take estrogen.

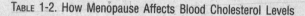

TABLE 1-2. How Menopause Affects Blood Cholesterol Levels

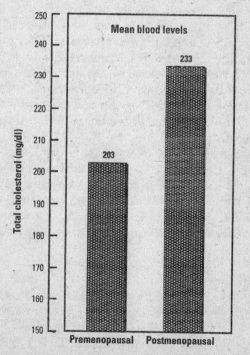

The menopause-related drop in estrogen also affects the ratios of artery-clogging low-density lipoproteins (LDL cholesterol), the "bad" cholesterol that raises your risk of heart disease, and high density lipoproteins (HDL cholesterol), the "good" cholesterol believed to protect against heart disease. For reasons that aren't clear yet, postmenopausal women are also more prone to develop atherosclerosis, or narrowing of the arteries—perhaps as a result of higher LDL and lower HDL cholesterol levels.

But not everyone is convinced that the drop in estrogen after menopause is the main culprit. One study involving 121,700 women found no increased cardiovascular risk associated with menopause. Other studies, including the famed Framingham Heart Study, have shown that premenopausal women who've had a hysterectomy are at much greater risk of developing heart disease than women who haven't had the surgery—*even when they haven't had their estrogen-producing ovaries removed*.

Whatever the reason for the rise in your risk of heart disease after menopause, one way to help offset the risk (as you will see in chapter 5) is to take hormone additive therapy. Numerous studies have shown that *women who take postmenopausal estrogens have about half the incidence of heart disease as women who don't take estrogen*.

Osteoporosis

We all lose bone mass as we age. Our research and that of other scientists has shown, however, that the drop in estrogen after menopause results in a more rapid loss of bone mass (see our study results in Table 1-3). If left untreated, this loss of bone mass weakens bones, making them more susceptible to fractures, a condition known as *osteoporosis*. Most vulnerable are the weight-bearing bones of the spine, which may collapse, resulting in compression fractures of the middle and lower back. Other susceptible bones are those of the hip and wrist. Osteoporosis is a major cause of disability and death in a woman's later years.

TABLE 1-3. How Menopause Affects Bone Density

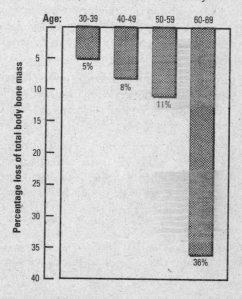

Fortunately, there's much you can do to slow (and possibly reverse) the rapid loss of bone mass associated with menopause. One thing you can do is take hormone additive therapy—particularly if you have low bone mass before you reach menopause.

Hysterectomy, Ovariectomy, and Surgical Menopause

Although hysterectomy (surgical removal of the uterus) is the second most commonly performed surgery in the United States (cesarean sections top the list), many women today are confused about just what a hysterectomy is—and whether they need to take postmenopausal hormone therapy after having this operation. Much of the confusion surrounding hysterectomy has to do with the terminology used to describe the operation. In fact, there are many different kinds of hysterectomy:

Hysterectomy or **simple hysterectomy**: The removal of the uterus and sometimes the attached Fallopian tubes. Your hormone-producing ovaries are left intact.

Total hysterectomy: Contrary to popular belief, this term does not mean that the ovaries are removed along with the uterus. Rather, it refers to the removal of the uterus and cervix. As with simple hysterectomy, you will still have your ovaries intact.

Subtotal or **partial hysterectomy:** These terms are used to describe the removal of the uterus above the cervix. The cervix and ovaries are left in place.

Oophorectomy (or ovariectomy): The medical term for the removal of one ovary. If you are premenopausal when you lose one ovary, the other ovary will take over, ovulating every month and producing estrogen and progesterone necessary to regulate your menstrual cycle. You will be able to bear children and you will experience a natural menopause as long as you have one functioning ovary.

Salpingo-oophorectomy: This means the loss of a Fallopian tube and an ovary on one side. Again, if only one ovary is removed before you experience a natural menopause, the other will compensate for the loss.

Bilateral oophorectomy: This term refers to the removal of both ovaries. If you have this operation before you experience a natural menopause, the procedure results in instantaneous, or "surgical" menopause, regardless of whether your uterus is left intact.

Bilateral salpingo-oophorectomy: The removal of both ovaries and Fallopian tubes. Again, premenopausal women who have this operation experience a surgical menopause.

Hysterectomy with bilateral salpingo-oophorectomy: This is the medical term for removal of the uterus, both Fallopian tubes, and both ovaries—what most women refer to as a "total" or "complete" hysterectomy. The operation results in surgical menopause among premenopausal women.

Many premenopausal women who have had a simple hysterectomy are surprised when, in their late forties and early fifties, they start experiencing hot flashes and other menopausal symptoms. One reason menopause may take you by surprise if you've had a hysterectomy in your childbearing years is that you no longer experience menstrual bleeding, or the telltale cessation of menstruation that alerts women with an intact uterus that menopause has, in fact, arrived. But because your ovaries remain intact and functioning, they will gradually produce less and less estrogen and progesterone and eventually, you may experience many of the same menopausal symptoms that women who undergo a natural menopause have. In fact, your menopause *will be* natural in every way but one: You won't experience the sometimes erratic menstrual cycles and bleeding patterns that lead up to menopause or the cessation of menstruation that lets you know that you have passed this biological milestone. If you've had a hysterectomy but still have your ovaries intact, the decision to take estrogen additive therapy is largely up to you.

Premenopausal women who have both ovaries removed are another story. Unlike women who go through a natural menopause and experience a gradual reduction in estrogen and progesterone over several years' time, these women undergo a sudden stoppage of the production of estrogen and progesterone often many years earlier than the natural decline in the production of these hormones would normally take place. For this reason, premenopausal women who have their ovaries removed often experience more and more severe symptoms of menopause, such as hot flashes, sleep disruptions, and vaginal dryness. What's more, premenopausal women who have an ovariectomy lose the natural protection these hormones provide the heart and bones many years earlier than if they had experienced a natural menopause. As a result, women who have had their ovaries removed are seven times more likely to develop coronary heart disease and are much more likely to develop osteoporosis at an early age than premenopausal women who don't have this operation. And while making life-style changes alone (exercising and eating a low-fat diet that's adequate in calcium, for instance) may be sufficient to protect many naturally menopausal women from heart disease and osteoporosis in their later years, *these measures usually aren't enough to offset the increased risk of heart disease and osteoporosis associated with a surgical menopause. You really should take estrogen, too.* In fact, this may be one of the only instances in which the commonly used term *estrogen replacement therapy* lives up to its name; *for premenopausal women who've had an ovariectomy, it is essential to replace the hormones that the ovaries normally would produce.*

The Importance of Regular Medical Checkups

If you're lucky, you won't even know you've experienced menopause until a year *after* your final menstrual period—the medical definition of menopause. Most women, however, will experience one or more of the classic symptoms, such as hot flashes and vaginal dryness, often *before* they've stopped menstruating. A minority will have symptoms severe enough to seek medical treatment.

Even more important than these nuisance symptoms are the "silent" changes in your body that often accompany menopause. As we've mentioned earlier, estrogen appears to have a protective effect on both your heart and your bones. When estrogen levels fall after menopause, you lose that built-in biological protection. As a result, your risk of heart disease and the bone-thinning disorder osteoporosis rises. For these reasons, even if you have *none* of the overt symptoms of menopause, or if symptoms are relatively mild, you should be monitored closely by your physician during the menopausal years to ensure that the silent changes don't take a toll on your health.

Ideally, you should have a premenopausal checkup between ages thirty-five and forty-five that includes (at the very least) a *lipid profile*—a test of your blood lipid (fat) levels (total cholesterol, LDL cholesterol, HDL cholesterol, and triglycerides), as well as a bone density screening test to determine how healthy your bones are *before* the effects of your menopause kick in. Once you reach menopause, you should have regular medical checkups throughout your menopausal years (ages fifty to sixty-five) to monitor the impact of your menopause on your heart and bones and to determine whether you might benefit from hormone additive therapy or other protective measures. (You'll find a complete description of recommended screening tests for pre- and postmenopausal women in our book *Menopause and Midlife Health*.)

The good news is that virtually *all* of the changes associated with the so-called Change of Life can be managed and their impact on your health and the quality of your life minimized. One of the most convenient ways to ensure a more comfortable menopause and good health in your later years is to take hormone additive therapy. In the chapters that follow, you'll learn more specifics about how estrogen affects your body and your health, and the ways in which hormone additive therapy can help make your menopause more manageable.

CHAPTER 2

🐚

Estrogen, Hot Flashes, and Other Menopausal Symptoms

Most of the symptoms of menopause are a direct result of low estrogen levels. Here's a look at some of the more common *vasomotor* symptoms, including the notorious hot flash, and how—for many women—estrogen can help.

Hot Flashes

Hot flashes are sometimes called the "badge of menopause" because they're so common among menopausal women. About 85 percent of perimenopausal women experience hot flashes (also known as hot flushes, night sweats, or vasomotor symptoms). Indeed, what was once chalked up as "all in your head" has finally become recognized as a real biological phenomenon that has a great impact on many women.

Hot flashes may begin *before* menopause and are a telltale sign that menopause is approaching. Most women, however, will experience hot flashes in the year or two after menopause. For the majority of women (65 percent), hot flashes occur over a period of from one to five years. Another 25 percent of women experience hot flashes over a period of six to ten years. A minority of women (10 percent) have hot flashes over a period of ten years or more.

For some women, hot flashes may be nothing more than an occasional fleeting sensation of warmth. Others may experience hourly waves of heat, drenching sweats, and a racing heart. Sleep may be disrupted several times a night by night sweats. The lack of sleep causes fatigue, irritability, and impaired memory. The sensations may last anywhere from thirty seconds up to thirty minutes. Some women experience as few as several hot flashes a year, while others with very severe hot flashes may suffer up to fifty per day. Daily hot flashes appear to be the norm.

You can expect to have more severe hot flashes if you've had a surgical menopause, at least for the first year after having your ovaries removed. This is probably because the drop in your level of estrogen is so abrupt. Surgically menopausal women are also more likely to suffer unrelenting hot flashes for years after menopause.

Hot flashes may feel worse in summer months or in hot, humid climates. And while many women report feeling hot flashes in the upper part of their body, the sensations can occur elsewhere as well.

It's hard to predict who will suffer hot flashes. It appears to be an equal opportunity phenomenon: Researchers have found no relation between hot flashes and employment status, social class, age, marital status, domestic workload, or number of children. They've also found no connection between hot flashes and a woman's age when she first begins menstruating, age at menopause, number of pregnancies, height, or medical problems. Indeed, the only factor that correlates with frequency of hot flashes in menopausal women is body weight: Women with hot flashes tend to weigh less and have less body fat than asymptomatic women.

Anatomy of a Hot Flash

To understand how a hot flash occurs, it helps to know a little bit about your body's temperature-regulating system. This remarkable system, which involves your skin and underlying fat tissues, your blood vessels, and central nervous system, allows your body to maintain a constant "core" temperature (that is, the temperature of the deep tissues of your body)—even when you are exposed to vast changes in the outside temperature. Except when you have a fever, your core temperature doesn't fluctuate more than one degree day in and day out.

The master controls, or thermostat, for your body's temperature-regulating system reside in the hypothalamus, the part of your brain that controls such basic needs as hunger and thirst, sex drive, and certain emotions. The hypothalamus contains large numbers of heat- and cold-sensitive nerve cells (neurons) that increase their activity when they sense a rise or fall in temperature. Still other neurons in the hypothalamus become excited in response to signals transmitted to the brain from cold and heat receptors in the skin and certain deep tissues in the body.

When the hypothalamus detects that your body temperature is too hot, it sends out signals to dilate the blood vessels, increasing blood flow to the skin. This allows excess body heat to be transferred to the skin and out of the body. The hypothalamus also activates sweat glands (located just under the skin), which help cool your body.

If the hypothalamus senses that your body temperature is too cold, it signals the blood vessels to constrict, which helps keep body heat from escaping. The hypothalamus also signals your body to generate more heat by shivering and by increasing your rate of metabolism.

A hot flash occurs when the hypothalamus somehow gets its signals mixed. Thinking your body temperature is too warm, it suddenly sets in motion the mechanisms to cool you off.

Studies have shown that immediately (five to sixty seconds) prior to the onset of a hot flash, many women experience a premonition, or *aura* of an impending hot flash. During this time, your heart rate and blood flow to the skin (particularly your hands and fingers) accelerate.

At the start of a hot flash, your skin becomes cold and clammy. Blood flow to your extremities increases four- to thirty-fold, and your heart rate continues to accelerate (from eight to sixteen beats more per minute than normal). Your finger temperature rises and you begin to sweat. As a result of these cooling mechanisms, your core body temperature drops, reaching a low about five to nine minutes after the onset of the hot flash. When your body temperature drops significantly, your blood vessels constrict, your metabolism increases, and you begin to shiver. This helps return your body temperature to normal.

What Causes a Hot Flash?

No one knows what causes this sudden, temporary downward resetting of the body's thermostat. It's natural to assume that estrogen plays a major role, since hot

flashes occur when estrogen levels drop around menopause. The abrupt onset of hot flashes after surgical removal of the ovaries and the relief of hot flashes with
estrogen therapy appear to support the argument.

But the exact role of estrogen is still a mystery:
Throughout your postmenopausal years, estrogen levels
remain low; yet some women never experience hot
flashes, while others have only sporadic hot flashes.
Preteenage girls have low estrogen levels and they
don't experience hot flashes. And hot-flash-like episodes have been reported during pregnancy, when estrogen levels are high. These facts, along with other
"circumstantial" evidence have led researchers to suspect that hot flashes are more a consequence of estrogen withdrawal rather than low estrogen levels. For
instance, obese women are less troubled than thin
women by hot flashes, probably because their increased
body fat converts androgens into estrogen, keeping estrogen levels somewhat higher. Plus, women who are
born without ovaries and who have never had normal
estrogen levels typically don't suffer hot flashes until
after they've been given estrogen therapy that is later
stopped.

Exactly how estrogen withdrawal triggers hot flashes
isn't known yet, either. Animal studies have shown that
estrogen increases the activity of heat-sensitive neurons
in the hypothalamus, and decreases the activity of cold-
sensitive neurons. Estrogen also increases blood flow
throughout your body. Estrogen works in several ways
to enhance the activity of epinephrine and norepinephrine, two neurotransmitters that also interact with the
hypothalamus and help control body temperature. These
neurotransmitters help control the dilation and contraction of blood vessels, particularly those in the fingers.

When a part of the hypothalamus in monkeys is stimulated with norepinephrine, they experience dilation of the blood vessels in their fingers and toes and a drop in their core body temperature similar to changes occurring in women during hot flashes. Estrogen withdrawal may somehow affect the activity of these neurotransmitters, thus triggering hot flashes.

Progesterone also appears to play a role in hot flashes. The rise in progesterone during the second half of the menstrual cycle raises the set point of the hypothalamus—and raises your body temperature. When you take progestogen (a synthetic form of progesterone), hot flashes may *feel* less severe because your body's thermostat has been adjusted to a higher setting.

Other hormones may be partly responsible for triggering hot flashes, as well. High levels of follicle-stimulating hormone (FSH) and luteinizing hormone (LH) were initially thought to play some role in triggering hot flashes. But hot flashes often decline or stop after menopause, in spite of continued high levels of these hormones. And hot flashes may persist even when LH and FSH levels are reduced by drugs such as danazol (Danocrin), a synthetic form of testosterone, which in the past has been used in the treatment of endometriosis.

On the other hand, when women who never had hot flashes take drugs that block gonadotropin releasing hormone (GnRH) receptors in the pituitary gland, they experience hot flashes for the first time. Although GnRH is not the immediate trigger of hot flashes, some people believe that it may somehow be involved in causing them.

The symptoms of menopausal hot flashes—visible

flushing of the neck and face, perspiration, goose bumps and shivering, and sleep disturbances such as insomnia and intermittent awakening—are also signs of narcotics withdrawal. This has led researchers to believe that beta endorphins and other *opiates*, naturally occurring narcotics in the body that are responsible for pain relief and feelings of euphoria, may play a role in hot flashes, too. Estrogen and progesterone have been found to alter the activity of these naturally occurring opioids. It's possible that lower levels of estrogen and progesterone cause a withdrawal of these substances from parts of the hypothalamus, triggering some of the same withdrawal symptoms that drug addicts experience.

Handling Hot Flashes: What You Can Do

If you experience mild to moderate hot flashes, there are several ways to increase your comfort level without resorting to drugs.

1. *Keep a record or diary of your hot flashes.* Hot flashes are not necessarily random occurrences that always take you by surprise. According to Ann Voda, R.N., Ph.D., at the University of Utah College of Nursing, many women find that certain substances or circumstances—a hot cup of coffee, for instance—act as triggers. Other common triggers are highly seasoned, spicy foods, hot beverages, and alcohol. By keeping a record once a month for a year, you may discover some of your own triggers, and may be better able to manage your hot flashes by avoiding those triggers.

2. *Wear layers of thin clothing that can be removed during a hot flash.* Clothes made of 100 percent cotton are best because they absorb moisture, dry quickly, and allow heat to escape.

3. *Keep your home and work environments cool.* As we mentioned earlier, a warm climate can make your hot flashes *feel* worse. Some women find that a hot environment acts as a trigger. To avoid this, set your office or home thermostat at 65 degrees Fahrenheit—lower if possible. Keep a hand fan in your purse and sit next to the air conditioner (or away from heat ducts) at meetings or social gatherings. To reduce nighttime awakenings, keep your room temperature at 65 degrees Fahrenheit or lower. Open the windows in winter. Turn on the air conditioner in summer.

4. *Avoid emotionally charged or stressful situations.* Emotional stress may trigger hot flashes in some women.

5. *When a hot flash occurs, run cold water over your wrists or splash water on your face to cool yourself off.* If possible, take a cold shower.

6. *Exercise regularly.* Regular physical activity may help alleviate hot flashes. Swedish researchers have found that among 634 women who had experienced a natural menopause and were not taking hormones, physically active women reported fewer and less severe hot flashes than inactive women. Only 6 percent of the active women studied had severe hot flashes, compared with 25 percent of the sedentary women. The researchers suspect that exercise helps counter hot flashes by raising the level and activity of beta endorphins in the body.

7. *Try biofeedback.* You may be able to train your body to (at least partially) override a hot flash through the use of biofeedback. Of eight women we trained in the use of biofeedback, all reported fewer and less se-

vere hot flashes after the training. Essentially, the women were told to "think warm" throughout the day to keep the thermostat in their bodies at a higher set point. At the onset of a hot flash, the women were instructed to "think cold" to help return their body temperature back to normal. Ask your physician or other health professional about biofeedback training.

Handling Hot Flashes: What Your Doctor Can Do

If your hot flashes are so severe that they regularly interfere with daily living and the quality of your life, estrogen is by far the most effective drug therapy available. Estrogen is more than 95 percent effective in relieving hot flashes.

If you have an intact uterus, you will have to take a progestogen, either cyclically or continuously, along with estrogen. But there's some evidence to suggest that progestogen helps relieve hot flashes, as well (see below). In fact, taking a combination of estrogen and progestogen may be even more effective than taking estrogen alone.

If you can't or don't want to take estrogen, your doctor has a variety of other drugs that can help ease hot flashes, although none are quite so effective as estrogen. These include

Progestogen: Researchers accidentally discovered that progestogen can be used to treat hot flashes when women with endometrial cancer who were taking progestogen also experienced relief of their hot flashes. The higher the dose of progestogen, the greater the relief. Like estrogen, you need to take progestogen for a couple of weeks before hot flashes abate, and up to four weeks before you experience maximum relief.

Progestogen may be useful for women who can't take estrogen. One type of progestogen, *megestrol acetate* (Megace), is often prescribed to help control hot flashes in women who have had breast cancer. But the drug may cause weight gain, irregular bleeding, abdominal bloating, breast tenderness, and mood changes. Progestogens may adversely affect blood lipid levels.

Androgens: These drugs are effective in controlling hot flashes when used alone or with estrogen. When used alone, however, higher doses may be needed, leading to more severe side effects, including growth of facial hair and a deepening voice.

Clonidine (Catapres): This drug, usually prescribed to lower blood pressure, also relieves hot flashes, but not as effectively as estrogen. No one is sure exactly how the drug works. Scientists know that it blocks the neurotransmitters epinephrine and norepinephrine and it appears to stabilize the temperature-regulating center of the hypothalamus. Clonidine may also block the dilation of blood vessels in the arms and legs, which occurs during a hot flash.

In the largest studies, clonidine reduced the frequency of hot flashes from 12 to 40 percent (depending on the dosage). However, higher doses were related to bothersome side effects, including dry mouth and dizziness. Clonidine works best when delivered via a skin patch worn on your shoulder and changed once a week.

Methyldopa (Aldomet), yet another blood pressure medication that works the same way as clonidine, appears to help relieve hot flashes, too. Studies have shown that methyldopa reduces the frequency of hot flashes by 20 percent compared with a placebo. With both of these drugs, however, side effects such as dry mouth, fatigue, and headache limit their use.

Other drugs: There's some evidence that the analgesic *naproxen* (Anaprox), a nonsteroidal anti-inflammatory agent, reduces hot flashes. Beta blockers, drugs used to treat high blood pressure and other heart problems, appear to be effective in treating hot flashes, as well, although these drugs are less effective in treating other menopausal symptoms, such as anxiety and insomnia.

Bellergal: This tranquilizer has been found to reduce the number and intensity of hot flashes by 50 percent among women who take it. No one's sure which of its ingredients, including phenobarbital, a potent tranquilizer, is responsible for its effectiveness. The drug is particularly effective if your most prominent symptom is perspiration. However, it may cause constipation and dry mouth in some users. As for the phenobarbital, the levels in Bellergal are not very high, so addiction is usually not a problem. The drug is a good choice for women with breast cancer, who are usually advised not to take estrogen. It may also be useful for postmenopausal women who suffer from migraine headaches.

Bellergal comes in time-released tablets that can be taken once before bedtime or, if hot flashes are severe, once in the morning and again at night.

Sleep Disruptions

A primary complaint of women with hot flashes is that their sleep is disrupted. For a while, experts believed these sleep disruptions were chiefly caused by night sweats. But studies have shown that sleep disturbances are not always a result of hot flashes, and not all hot flashes disrupt sleep. Indeed, while most hot flashes are associated with waking episodes, 40 percent of waking episodes are not associated with hot flashes.

Taking over-the-counter or prescription sleeping pills won't necessarily guarantee you a good night's sleep, since these medications do nothing to treat the underlying problem. What's more, these drugs reduce the amount of dream sleep (also known as rapid-eye-movement, or REM sleep), a certain amount of which is needed to help you feel well-rested and mentally alert.

For occasional sleeplessness, specialists in sleep disorders recommend that you first try to improve your sleep habits or "sleep hygiene" by changing your lifestyle and environment. This approach includes the following common-sense tips:

   1. *Keep to a sleep schedule.* Go to bed at the same time every night and get up at the same time every morning. Maintaining a fairly regular schedule helps set your body clock so that your sleep and wake times become routine. If you haven't fallen asleep within thirty minutes, or if you wake up in the middle of the night and can't get back to sleep, get up and do something relaxing, such as reading or sewing, until you feel sleepy. Don't lie in bed tossing and turning.
   2. *Control your sleep environment.* Sleep in a darkened room. If window shades don't make the room dark enough, wear an eye covering. Block out noise as much as possible by wearing ear plugs, if necessary. Or mask the noise by running an air conditioner or fan. Keep the

room cool, too. It's hard to sleep when you're uncomfortably warm.

3. *Get regular exercise.* Daily workouts have been shown to be extremely effective in tiring out the body and preparing it for a good night's sleep. Don't exercise shortly before bedtime, however. Late-night workouts can overstimulate your body, contributing to insomnia.

4. *Use your bed for sleep (and lovemaking) only.* Don't work, eat, or watch television in bed.

5. *Avoid caffeinated drinks and foods late in the day.* Caffeine is a well-recognized stimulant. If you're having trouble sleeping, stay away from coffee, tea, caffeinated soft drinks, or other caffeine-containing foods and beverages in the late afternoon or evening.

If menopause-related insomnia is severe enough to interfere with daily living, the best treatment is estrogen therapy. Women who take estrogen fall asleep faster, sleep longer, have fewer episodes of wakefulness, and have more periods of dream sleep than women who take a placebo. (If you're using estrogen therapy to help relieve sleep, you should take your estrogen just before bedtime. This way, blood estrogen levels will peak during the night and help you sleep better.)

Of course, sleep disturbances and early morning awakenings are also signs of major depression. If you suffer from sleep disturbances, you should undergo a complete physical *and* psychological evaluation to rule out other possible causes.

Emotional Changes (the "Menopausal Syndrome")

Although many women fear that menopause will make them "go crazy" or "fall apart," new research is challenging this long-held belief. Recent studies have found no increased incidence of depression among menopausal women. And rather than having regrets about losing their ability to bear children, most women today express *relief* that they don't have to worry about contraception anymore.

Nevertheless, a minority of women may experience emotional ups and downs related to the hormonal changes of menopause. Mood changes such as irritability, depression, insomnia, impaired memory, and crying jags frequently precede and follow menopause. In many instances, these changes are "hormone-related."

How can hormones influence your mood? To begin with, irritability, impaired memory, and anxiety are typical signs of chronic sleep disturbances—particularly dream sleep (See "sleep disruptions," above), and hot flashes and night sweats often disrupt sleep. Hormones in themselves appear to affect your mood, as well. Several studies have shown that estrogen and a combination of estrogen and androgen (the "male" hormone testosterone) appear to have a "mental-tonic" effect on women who take them. The feeling of well-being associated with these hormones may stem from the hormones' direct effect on the brain: Estrogen receptors have been found in parts of the brain that govern emotions, including the hypothalamus. Estrogen may also affect a number of different neurotransmitters that have been tied to feelings of depression and elation. For instance, estrogen is believed to reduce levels of the brain

chemical *monoamine oxidase* (MAO). The lower levels
of MAO in turn *increase* certain mood-altering chemicals in the brain, including norepinephrine and serotonin. (Certain depressions have been associated with
decreased levels of these brain chemicals, especially
norepinephrine.) Estrogen appears to *increase* levels of
other brain chemicals, notably the more biologically active "free" tryptophan, a precursor of serotonin.

Whatever the mechanism that causes mood swings
and other psychological symptoms, women whose
symptoms are *hormone-related* often find relief with estrogen therapy. Aside from the "mental-tonic" effect
that estrogen has, it also helps you sleep better at night
and in this way may improve your sense of well-being.

Of course, hormones won't help women who are suffering from true clinical depression or other serious
psychological problems. Also, trouble on the homefront
or at work could trigger bouts of insomnia, irritability,
depression, and mood swings, which won't be influ-
enced by hormone therapy. Obviously, then, it's important to make the distinction between hormone-related
symptoms and those that are not related to hormones.
But this is often not easy to do. You should start by un-
dergoing a thorough physical and psychological evaluation. We make a point of asking, "How are things at
home?" during each patient's physical examination to
ensure that other possible causes of these symptoms
aren't overlooked.

If the cause of the symptoms is still not clear after a
complete medical and psychological evaluation, you
may want to try taking hormones. If you feel better
once you start hormone therapy, you simply continue
the treatment. If your symptoms are the same or become worse after taking hormone therapy, this is a sign

that you and your physician should look for another cause—and treatment regimen.

Headaches

Many women who suffer from "menstrual migraines" (migraine headaches that coincide with hormonal changes such as menstruation, ovulation, and use of birth control pills) may find that their headaches improve or remit during menopause. Such headaches are believed to be triggered by fluctuating estrogen levels—particularly a drop in estrogen after a period of several days' exposure to high levels of estrogen. The constant, lower levels of estrogen after menopause may help explain why headaches improve.

For reasons we don't fully understand, migraine headaches continue and even accelerate for some women after menopause. These women may be helped by continuous estrogen therapy. (The estrogen patch works particularly well.) Estrogen raises levels of pain-relieving opioids in the brain and stabilizes certain mood-altering catecholamines (dopamine and serotonin), which may be why estrogen often eliminates migraines.

Estrogen doesn't *always* relieve menopausal migraines. Some women may find that estrogen actually makes their migraines worse. If after trying different types of estrogen therapy, your headaches have *worsened*, you may have to try a different treatment approach. Ask your physician about other possible therapies.

For the most part, women who suffer "menopausal migraines" have a long history of migraines. If you suddenly begin experiencing severe, debilitating migraine-like headaches after menopause, you should undergo a complete physical examination to rule out other possible causes. Often, migraine headaches that develop after menopause are *not* hormone-related.

Should You Take Estrogen for Your Menopausal Symptoms?

For a majority of women, menopausal symptoms are quite manageable without any medical intervention. Do you need hormone additive therapy? Since there are no standardized medical tests that objectively measure many menopause-related symptoms, such as hot flashes, we've found that the best judge as to whether you need treatment is *you*. Fill out the Menopausal Symptoms Questionnaire on page 145 to help determine which menopause-related symptoms you may be experiencing and which may require treatment.

If you experience emotional symptoms, such as mood swings, crying jags, or depression, your physician may recommend that you also undergo a psychological evaluation. This may involve being interviewed by a qualified counselor or therapist (ask your regular doctor for a recommendation) or simply filling out a standardized questionnaire.

If you and your doctor determine that your symptoms are severe enough to interfere with daily living, and if the self-help measures discussed in this chapter don't help, you should seriously consider taking hormone additive therapy, which is one of the most effective ways of relieving these symptoms.

CHAPTER 3

❧

Can Estrogen Improve
Your Sex Life?

You've probably heard rumors that menopause will put an end to your sex life. Is it true? While sexual problems—for men and women—*do* tend to escalate in the menopausal years (only 18 percent of women in their twenties and thirties report having a sexual problem; the number rises to 28 percent in women over age fifty), there's no reason why you *can't* have a fulfilling sex life after menopause and throughout your later years.

There are a number of reasons for the decline in sexual activity and the increase in sexual problems as couples grow older. For women, one of the most common problems—painful intercourse (*dyspareunia*)—arises from changes in the vagina related to low estrogen levels after menopause, and can be easily treated with estrogen cream. Let's take a closer look at some of the physical changes that affect you *and* your partner. With a little knowledge, a lot of reassurance, and medical treatment, if necessary, these changes don't have to bring an end to your sex life.

Physical Changes in Men and Women

Sexual problems can arise at any time during your life. (Remember the first time you had sex?) One reason why older men and women have more problems is that they both undergo physiological changes that can make lovemaking more difficult. For instance, men generally take longer to achieve an erection as they grow older, and the erection may be less full. The amount of sperm decreases with age, as well. Sometimes, no semen is ejaculated at all. Other times, men may experience *retrograde ejaculation*, in which semen is ejaculated back into the bladder, where it is later passed in the urine. No harm occurs in any of these situations, and they need not interfere with the enjoyment of sex for you and your partner.

Women, too, undergo subtle (and sometimes not so subtle) physical changes that may affect their sex life. For example, while you won't lose your ability to have an orgasm as you grow older, the number of involuntary contractions of the uterus during orgasm decreases. As you grow older, the clitoris retracts and shrinks faster, after orgasm, too. But these changes should in no way detract from sexual satisfaction.

Remember, too, that it's perfectly normal for a woman *not* to have an orgasm during intercourse. In fact a majority of women don't. This is because the vagina simply doesn't have an abundance of nerve endings. The clitoris, on the other hand, does contain numerous sensitive nerve endings that respond to direct stimulation. Most women need direct stimulation of the clitoris to achieve orgasm. Telling your partner this, or even stimulating the clitoris yourself can often solve a major sexual problem.

Some women find that applying a small amount of testosterone cream to the clitoris helps it respond to stimulation and enhances the quality of an orgasm. This, in turn, may also stimulate your sex drive by making orgasms more intense and enjoyable.

The most dramatic physical changes for women usually occur ten to fifteen years after menopause. Let's look more closely at how menopause can affect your sexuality.

Vaginal Dryness

Changes in the vagina resulting from low estrogen after menopause are likely to have the biggest impact on your sex life. As estrogen levels fall during menopause, estrogen-sensitive tissues in the vagina respond. The outer folds of the vagina shrink, causing the skin to sag and become dry. Capillaries in the vaginal walls shrink, as well, reducing blood flow and nutrients to these tissues. The vaginal lining (epithelium) becomes pale and thin, making the vagina susceptible to irritation and infection. Over many years' time, these changes decrease the thickness of the epithelium, increase the pH (acid-base balance) of the vagina, change the bacterial flora in your vagina, and decrease blood flow to the vagina. As a result, many postmenopausal women experience vaginal dryness or a discharge, and vaginal itching and burning—a condition known as *atrophic vaginitis*.

As a result of these changes, you may experience delayed or reduced vaginal secretions during sexual stimulation. Whereas it may have taken a minute for your vagina to become lubricated at age twenty-five, now it may take you fifteen minutes or longer. Lack of lubrication can make lovemaking painful, a condition physicians call *dyspareunia*. Some women may even bleed after intercourse as a result of trauma to the fragile vaginal walls. You may first notice the itching and burning of atrophic vaginitis only after sexual encounters. Later, you may notice a dry feeling in the vagina throughout the day.

Low estrogen levels also may affect your urinary tract (see chapter 4), which can result in urinary frequency or urgency, and sometimes loss of bladder control (urinary incontinence). Some women may be embarrassed about losing control of their bladder during intercourse.

These may seem like minor irritations. But they can have major consequences: When symptoms interfere with sexual performance, they can lead to a decrease in desire and self-esteem, and to an increase in anxiety. In a study we conducted along with Gloria Bachmann, M.D., at the University of Medicine and Dentistry of New Jersey in New Brunswick, women complaining of vaginal dryness reported a 72 percent decrease in sexual frequency, a 71 percent decrease in desire, and a 78 percent decrease in sexual satisfaction and arousal.

While it's natural to feel anxiety about having sexual intercourse when you're afraid it may hurt, anxiety can actually decrease blood flow to the vagina, making matters even worse. If lines of communication shut down (as they often do when sexual problems arise), your partner may interpret your lack of sexual initiative as a lack of sexual desire for him. Or your partner may worry so much about hurting you that he loses interest in sex himself, thus fueling a vicious cycle of sexual problems for both partners. A third of the women in our study reported that vaginal dryness had an effect on their partner as well. Indeed, the most common reason postmenopausal women at our clinic give for seeking estrogen therapy is not the physical pain associated with intercourse, but the psychological ramifications it has on their relationship.

Coping with Vaginal Dryness: What You Can Do

There are several things you can do to lessen the impact of vaginal dryness on your sex life.

1. *Keep sexually active.* Surprisingly, one way to keep vaginal walls healthy is to stay sexually active. Studies have found that women who engage in sexual activity at least once a week have significantly lower pH values and maintain better vaginal health than those who don't. This is because sexual arousal does produce some natural lubrication, chiefly by increasing blood flow to the vagina, which aids in the secretion of lubricating fluid through the vaginal lining. (The vagina has no glands.) Any sexual activity—even self-stimulation—helps improve blood flow and keep tissues supple.

2. *Take your time.* When you do make love, do so in a relaxed, unhurried atmosphere. Recognize that it may take longer for your vagina to become lubricated. Sometimes, taking a warm bath before lovemaking helps to relax your muscles and stimulate vaginal secretions.

3. *Use a lubricant.* Some women use a water-based lubricant, such as K-Y Jelly, particularly during intercourse. However, these lubricants don't provide long-lasting relief of vaginal symptoms, nor do they appear to lower vaginal pH.

A promising new lubricant called Replens contains

the compound *polycarbophil*, which appears to work even better than water-based lubricants. Indeed, the new lubricant may be almost as effective as estrogen in lowering vaginal pH and restoring a more normal vaginal milieu. In the study we conducted along with Dr. Gloria Bachmann, we compared the effects of Replens and a water-based lubricant on women complaining of vaginal itching, burning, irritation, pressure, and dyspareunia. While both the water-based lubricant and the polycarbophil-based moisturizer improved vaginal moisture, only the polycarbophil moisturizer lowered pH, increased the quantity of vaginal secretions, and decreased the fragility of the vaginal lining. And while more than 80 percent of the women in the study reported improved symptoms with nonhormonal therapy, 61 percent preferred the new vaginal moisturizer. One application of Replens lasts from forty-eight to seventy-two hours, so you don't have to use this type of lubricant just before intercourse or every time you have intercourse.

Whatever you do, *don't* use petroleum jelly as a lubricant; it actually causes more drying of the vaginal lining.

4. *Change the sexual script.* There's no rule dictating that making love means having intercourse. If intercourse is just too painful, try other means of stimulation, such as oral sex or self-stimulation.

How Estrogen Can Help Relieve Vaginal Dryness
Postmenopausal estrogen is simply the most effective treatment for vaginal dryness. In fact, postmenopausal estrogen can actually *reverse* many of the menopause-related changes in the vaginal tissues. Estrogen creams increase blood flow to the vagina and thicken the vagi-

nal epithelium (lining). Estrogen also improves the acid-base (pH) balance of the vagina, which may reduce your risk of developing vaginal infections.

A note of caution: You should *not* use vaginal estrogen creams as a lubricant before having intercourse. At least one report in the medical literature traced a man's breast enlargement to his wife's liberal use of estrogen creams. We subsequently conducted a study to see how well estrogen creams were absorbed through a man's penis and into his bloodstream. Study participants applied estrogen creams to the penis, and blood samples were taken hourly for six hours, and again twenty-four hours later, to monitor estrogen levels in the men's bloodstream. After two hours, blood estrogen (estrone) levels more than doubled. Levels of the male hormone androgen fell by more than 50 percent, as well. After twenty-four hours, however, the men's blood hormone levels had returned to normal.

We still don't know what impact, if any, a woman's use of estrogen creams will have on her partner's health. But given the penis's ability to absorb estrogen, it's probably better *not* to use estrogen creams as a lubricant.

Sexual Desire

It's not clear what effect—if any—the hormone changes of menopause have on a woman's sexual desire. Some women feel greater sexual desire because their children are out of the house, or because they no longer have to worry about unwanted pregnancy. Others may experience a temporary decrease in desire as a result of bothersome menopausal symptoms, such as hot flashes, fatigue, and irritability.

Interestingly, the male sex hormone testosterone is probably more important for maintaining sexual desire after menopause than estrogen. High levels of testosterone have been linked to greater feelings of desire and more frequent sexual fantasies among postmenopausal women who take them (see page 119). With that in mind, you'll be happy to know about the results of our 1982 study on menopause and aging. We found that while total testosterone levels *do* decline somewhat after a natural menopause, levels of the more biologically active *free testosterone* remain essentially unchanged by menopause. *So there appears to be no biological reason why sexual desire should decline after menopause.*

If you do feel a decrease in sexual desire after menopause, particularly because of bothersome menopausal symptoms, be sure to reassure your partner that your lack of sexual desire isn't a lack of desire for *him*. Often, when troublesome menopausal symptoms are treated with hormone additive therapy (or an alternative therapy), sexual interest and satisfaction are restored.

Should You Take Estrogen to Keep Sexually Active?

If you experience vaginal itching, irritation, or pain during intercourse, you should report these symptoms to your physician without delay. Your doctor will first rule out other possible causes of vaginitis, such as infection. He or she can also perform a pH balance test using secretions from the side walls of the vagina. A pH of less than 4.5 is considered normal; any values above 5 mean the vaginal pH has become too alkaline—a sign of atrophic vaginitis. Finally, your doctor may perform a test to determine the vagina's *maturation index*, in which a small sample of cells is gently removed from the side walls of the vagina (much like a Pap smear) and viewed under a microscope to determine the percentage of *parabasal cells*. If 20 percent or more of the cells are this type, a diagnosis of atrophic vaginitis will be made. Once your doctor has made a definitive diagnosis, the decision to use estrogen cream is up to you.

Keep in mind that while estrogen cream can make intercourse more comfortable, and in this way may increase your desire to have sex, estrogen in itself probably won't increase your sexual appetite. Using an estrogen cream won't necessarily solve long-standing sexual problems or those complicated by other factors, such as chronic illness, either. If problems persist even after estrogen creams (or alternative measures) relieve the physical discomfort caused by atrophic vaginitis, you and your partner may want to consider seeing a counselor or sex therapist. Ask your doctor for a referral.

CHAPTER 4

❧

Estrogen and Urinary
Symptoms

The bladder and urethra develop from the same tissues as the vagina in the growing embryo, so you can see how the hormonal changes of menopause could have an effect on these tissues. As with the vagina, the cells lining the urinary tract respond to hormonal changes by becoming thinner and more easily inflamed. These changes in your urinary tract may increase your risk of developing a urinary tract infection. Inflamed tissues of the urinary tract may also cause such symptoms as an increase in the number of times you urinate, a sudden urge to urinate, and low abdominal pressure; a condition known as *urethral syndrome. Urinary stress incontinence* (loss of bladder control when you sneeze, cough, or laugh) may worsen after menopause, too, as the hormonal changes associated with menopause cause the supporting ligaments surrounding the urethra to relax and the pressure in the urethra to decrease. Vaginal estrogen creams can often improve these problems and, in some women, may alleviate them altogether.

Urinary Tract Infections

Because of their anatomy, women are more prone than men to develop bacterial infections of the urethra *(urethritis)*, bladder *(cystitis)*, and, if left untreated, the kidney *(pyelocystitis)*. Your urethra (the tube leading from the bladder to the outside of the body) is much shorter than a man's, and is situated close to the vagina and rectum (see Figure 4-1). Bacteria from the vagina may work its way into the urethra during intercourse. Or if you clean yourself from back to front after a bowel movement, instead of from front to back, you may inadvertently spread bacteria from the rectum to the urethra. Indeed, the most common bacterial culprit is *E. coli*, found in the colon. Having a new sexual partner or using a diaphragm may increase the risk of infection. Women with diabetes, those with a kidney obstruction or suppressed immune system, and pregnant women are also more prone to developing a urinary tract infection.

As we pointed out earlier, the lower estrogen levels associated with menopause cause the lining of the urinary tract *(urothelium)* to thin out in much the same way as a lack of estrogen affects the lining of the vaginal walls. These changes in the urinary tract may increase your risk of developing a urinary tract infection after menopause. Normally, the mucus-producing glands in the lower portion of the urethra (the *periurethral glands*) trap bacteria and secrete bacteria-fighting immune cells. These safeguards help prevent the infection from ascending to the bladder. However, the menopause-related change in the urethral lining weakens the built-in biological protection you have.

Figure 4-1. The Female Urinary Tract

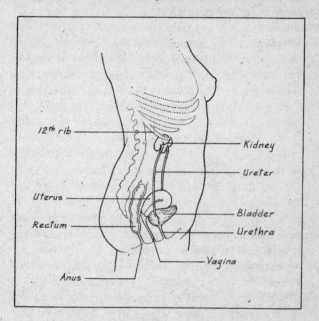

Low estrogen levels may also cause a decline in an important "mechanical barrier" to the spread of bacteria. Along the length of the urethra are muscle fibers that help control the flow of urine from the bladder. The muscles are thickest midway up the urethra, where they create a "pressure zone" that helps contain bacteria in the lower part of the urethra. When estrogen levels fall after menopause, blood flow to the area decreases and muscle tone may weaken, causing urethral pressure to decline and allowing bacteria to more easily migrate up to the bladder.

Finally, prolapse of the bladder, or *cystocele*, is more common among older women. This may make it more difficult for you to completely empty your bladder, and the residual pool of urine in the bladder may form a nidus for bacteria to multiply.

Symptoms include a frequent need to urinate (throughout the day *and* night) or a strong urge even when there's no need, lower abdominal pressure, pain upon urination, and possibly blood in the urine. Infections may also stimulate urge incontinence, in which you leak a small amount of urine before you have a chance to get to the bathroom.

You should take urinary tract infections seriously. While many infections remain localized in the lower urethra, an untreated infection can travel to the bladder and up the ureters to the kidneys, possibly leading to permanent kidney damage. *Never* try to self-treat a urinary tract infection with cranberry juice or other home remedies. If you have symptoms of an infection, see your physician, who will perform a few diagnostic tests to confirm your suspicions. A simple urinalysis, in which chemically treated paper is dipped into a sample of your urine, can detect white and red blood cells, possible signs of infection. Because the type of bacteria causing the infection could influence the type of drugs used to treat it, your physician may also want to perform a urine culture, in which a sample of your urine is sent to a laboratory and the bacteria in it are grown in a special culture medium.

If you have a urinary tract infection, your doctor will prescribe antibiotics to kill the bacteria causing your symptoms, and possibly a vaginal anti-yeast cream or suppository to prevent a secondary vaginal yeast infection.

Preventing Urinary Tract Infections

There are several measures you can take to reduce your chances of developing a urinary tract infection.

1. *Drink plenty of fluids.* Ideally, you should drink a glass of water every two to three hours to flush out the bladder.

2. *Urinate "when nature calls" and empty your bladder completely.* Holding your urine for long periods of time may encourage infection. If you have a cystocele (prolapse of the bladder), you can help empty the bladder by inserting a finger into your vagina and pushing up on the front of the vaginal wall as you urinate.

3. *Practice "safe sex."* You should urinate just before and right after having intercourse to help wash any wayward bacteria out of the urethra. During intercourse, avoid undue pressure on the front of the vaginal wall, which could irritate the urethra and cause a bout of Honeymoon cystitis. If your partner enters you from behind, take care not to sweep bacteria from the rectum up to the urethra. If you are prone to developing Honeymoon cystitis, you may want to consider taking a preventive dose of antibiotics after intercourse (for instance, Macrodantin or Septra).

4. *After urination or a bowel movement* always *wipe from front to back.* Regularly washing the area with a bidet or "peri" bottle (a small plastic squirt bottle filled with water that's usually recommended for cleaning the perineum in the weeks after childbirth) may further reduce the risk of infection.

5. *Change tampons and menstrual pads often to discourage the growth of bacteria.*

6. *Ask your physician to test the pH (acid-base balance) of your vagina.* If your physician finds that your vaginal pH is above 4.5, this usually means that the urethral pH is elevated as well. In that case, you may want to consider using a vaginal estrogen cream.

7. *Take your symptoms seriously.* If you develop symptoms of a urinary tract infection, report them to your doctor. *Don't* try to treat the symptoms yourself.

The Urethral Syndrome and Trigonitis

This syndrome is very common among postmenopausal women, and is often misdiagnosed as recurrent urinary tract infections. The symptoms—frequency of urination, urgency, and lower abdominal pressure—are similar to those for bladder infections, with one exception: You may experience little or no pain upon urination.

Urethral syndrome probably has more than one cause, but low estrogen levels after menopause most definitely contribute to the condition. The lining of the urethra contains estrogen receptors and, when estrogen levels fall after menopause, it may become pale and thin, sometimes causing inflammation. (Note: Even women taking oral estrogen can develop these symptoms.)

Regardless of the cause, a correct diagnosis is essential for treating the condition. Your physician will first perform a urinalysis and a urine culture to check for signs of a urinary tract infection. (Your doctor may also perform urethral cultures to rule out the sexually transmitted diseases *gonorrhea* and *chlamydia*, which may not be detected with a standard urine culture. This involves gently inserting a cotton swab in the urethra and sending a sample of cells to a laboratory to be grown in a culture dish.)

Your doctor will also perform a physical exam to screen for any physical abnormalities that may be causing symptoms of low abdominal pressure, such as prolapse of the bladder *(cystocele)*, rectum *(rectocele)*, uterus, or intestines *(enterocele)*. He or she may also perform a "pressure test" by inserting a finger into your vagina and pressing forward on the vaginal wall (where the urethra is located) to see if your symptoms can be reduplicated. Another test that may be recommended is *uroflowmetry*, which helps determine the average amount of urinary flow and the time it takes you to urinate. This test is usually performed by sitting on a specially designed chair and urinating into a bowl attached to a pressure sensing device.

Your physician may then perform a *urethroscopy* to look inside the urethra. The test is performed while you are lying on an examining table with your feet in the stirrups. Using a small insulin syringe (without the needle), your doctor will first insert a local anesthetic jelly into the urethra. The urethroscope, a thin lighted tube, will then be carefully inserted into the urethra to check for visible signs of inflammation, polyps, or other abnormalities of the urethral lining and trigone. The test takes from five to ten minutes. The amount of discomfort you experience depends on the amount of inflammation present.

Just as there are many possible causes of urethral syndrome, there are numerous ways to treat it. Your doctor will treat the most probable cause(s), depending on the results of your diagnostic workup.

Antibiotics. If your doctor suspects or finds evidence of an infection such as *chlamydia*, he or she may first prescribe antibiotics (tetracycline, doxycycline, or erythromycin) for two weeks.

Vaginal estrogen creams. If your symptoms persist even after taking antibiotics, or if a urethroscopic examination shows you have urethral syndrome stemming from low estrogen levels, a vaginal estrogen cream may be prescribed. (Estrogen creams placed in the vagina are well-absorbed by the urethral tissues.) Some studies show that up to half of all postmenopausal women who suffer from urethral syndrome improve after taking estrogen. Estrogen helps thicken the urethral lining and improves blood flow to the area. Estrogen also improves urethral pressure, all of which result in better bladder control.

Urethral dilations. This procedure, which can be performed right in your doctor's office, is believed to work in several different ways: The dilators massage and open up inflamed or infected urethral glands, helping to increase lubrication. Dilations may also massage the mucous membranes of the urethra, stretch the underlying tissues, and relieve stenosis (narrowing of the urethra), helping to improve the flow of urine.

The procedure itself takes less than ten minutes. During the procedure, you lie on an examining table with your feet in the stirrups. Our method involves inserting a small amount of estrogen cream into the urethra to act as a lubricant and to directly treat the inflamed urethral tissues with estrogen. The physician will then slowly insert and remove a series of metal dilators into the urethra, starting with the smallest in diameter and progressing to increasingly larger diameters until either the largest in diameter is inserted or you experience discomfort. After the procedure, more estrogen cream and possibly cortisone is inserted into the urethra to reduce inflammation. The procedure is performed once a week for three consecutive weeks. To help prevent a secondary infection, your doctor may recommend that you take an antibiotic (for instance, Macrodantin) every day for a month while you undergo urethral dilations. You should also use an estrogen cream for three months to a year after the dilations, and take an antibiotic after intercourse.

If symptoms recur after your treatment is over, your physician may recommend that you use a vaginal estrogen cream for up to one year.

Stress Urinary Incontinence

Stress incontinence is a type of urinary incontinence (temporary loss of bladder control) that typically occurs only during the stress of a sudden increase in abdominal pressure, such as when you cough, sneeze, lift things, laugh, or climb stairs. You may notice a loss of small to moderate amounts of urine—particularly when you cough, laugh, or sneeze—during the day, and little or no leakage at night.

Stress incontinence is caused by reduced urethral pressure and is usually associated with weakened or damaged supporting ligaments around the bladder neck. Although genetics, the trauma of childbirth, obesity, weak pelvic floor muscles, and cigarette smoking may all contribute to stress incontinence, the drop in estrogen levels associated with menopause can often make the problem worse. Low estrogen levels may decrease the strength and tone of the smooth muscle of the urethra needed to maintain urethral pressure.

If you experience *any* kind of involuntary urine leakage, see your doctor, who can offer a number of diagnostic tests to help make an accurate diagnosis. If you have genuine stress incontinence, surgery is usually required to correct the problem. Your doctor may recommend that you use a vaginal estrogen cream for a month or two before your surgery, which improves blood flow and urethral pressure, ultimately helping to ensure a better surgical outcome. (Note: Using estrogen cream alone is *not* sufficient enough to treat the problem; surgery is almost always required.)

Preventing Stress Urinary Incontinence: Advice for Menopausal Women with No Symptoms

There are some steps you can take to help *prevent* urinary stress incontinence.

1. *Have your physician test the strength of the pelvic floor muscle prior to menopause and afterward.* If sophisticated testing equipment isn't available for an objective measurement, your physician can simply insert a finger into your vagina and rectum and have you squeeze the muscle.

2. *If you are not using a vaginal estrogen cream, ask your physician to test the pH of your vagina during your annual examination.* If the pH is above 4.5, use a vaginal estrogen cream (half an applicatorful once or twice a week) as a preventive measure. Remember, estrogen improves blood flow to the area and may help maintain the tone of the urethra.

3. *Don't wait for your pelvic floor muscle to break down.* Exercise your right to remain continent by exercising the pelvic floor muscle every day. Perform the pelvic floor exercises (described below) daily until they increase and maintain the strength of the circumvaginal muscle.

Pelvic Floor Exercises

There is solid evidence that weak pelvic floor muscles contribute to stress urinary incontinence and possibly other types of incontinence. The pelvic floor muscle (also known as the *circumvaginal muscle*) is the main support of the pelvic organs (see Figure 4-2). Like any other muscle in the body, it needs to be regularly conditioned to maintain its strength and tone. In short, you either "use it or lose it."

FIGURE 4-2. Anatomy of the Female Pelvic Region

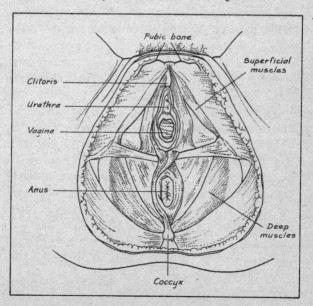

Pubic bone

Superficial muscles

Clitoris

Urethra

Vagina

Anus

Deep muscles

Coccyx

To locate the circumvaginal muscle, sit on the toilet, spread your legs apart and begin urinating. See if you can stop and start the flow of urine without moving your legs. If you can stop and start the stream, you are using the circumvaginal muscle. If you don't succeed the first time, keep trying until you have identified it.

Pelvic floor exercises can be performed any time, anywhere, in a seated or standing position. First contract the circumvaginal muscle and hold it for as long as you can, working your way up to eight to ten seconds. Then relax the muscle and repeat the exercise. Start with a set of fifteen contractions a day, adding ten more contractions per session each week until you can complete thirty-five to forty contractions per day.

A good way to remember to do your pelvic floor exercises is to exercise in the morning when you wake up, during certain daily activities, or before going to bed at night. In a week or two, you should begin to notice improved control. If you do not notice improvement after several weeks, consult your physician for further evaluation.

Another option for increasing the strength of the pelvic floor muscles is to use pelvic muscle training weights. A set of weights contains five vaginal cones that resemble tampons (including a string to remove them) ranging from twenty to seventy grams in weight. During a typical training program, you place the smallest weight in the vagina and wear it for ten to fifteen minutes two times a day. You must use your circumvaginal muscle to hold the weight in the vagina; otherwise, it will fall out. You begin by wearing the weight while you are seated, then graduate to a standing position. When you can hold the weight in place even as you cough or laugh, you are ready to progress to the next size weight.

The pelvic floor weights, called Femina Pelvic Muscle Training Weights, are manufactured by the Dacomed Corporation in Minneapolis, Minnesota. A set of five weights cost $99.00. If you are interested in ordering a set, ask your physician or call Dacomed's toll-free number: 800-328-1103.

CHAPTER 5

❧

Estrogen and Your Heart

We often think of heart disease as a "man's" illness. But cardiovascular disease is the leading cause of death for women, too. Because women are "protected" by estrogen before menopause, the prevalence of cardiovascular disease lags behind that of men by about a decade. However, by about age seventy, the rate in men and women is about the same. In terms of its absolute effect on women's health, cardiovascular disease is a primary concern: *Almost half of all deaths among women in the United States are a result of cardiovascular disease.*

In this chapter, you'll learn about the various ways in which estrogen helps protect women from cardiovascular disease—and how postmenopausal women can prolong their protection by taking hormone additive therapy. But first, you'll need a basic understanding of cardiovascular disease and how it develops.

How Heart Disease Develops

Cardiovascular disease is a broad term describing many different problems with the heart and circulatory system. One of the most worrisome for women in

56

FIGURE 5-1. How Plaque Forms in an Artery

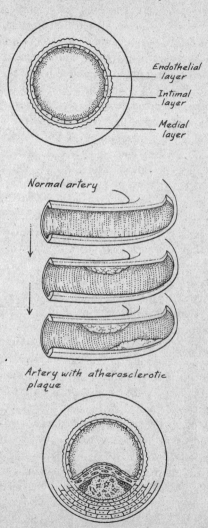

Endothelial
layer

Intimal
layer

Medial
layer

Normal artery

Artery with atherosclerotic
plaque

midlife is *coronary heart disease*. Coronary heart disease occurs when the arteries that supply oxygen and nutrients to the heart muscle become narrowed or blocked. Some thickening and hardening of the arteries is a part of normal aging, a process called *arteriosclerosis*. Far more insidious, however, is *atherosclerosis*, a type of arteriosclerosis in which deposits of fatty substances, cholesterol, cellular waste products, calcium, and *fibrin* (the tough fibers of a blood clot) build up on the inner lining of the artery, forming a hard *plaque* (see Figure 5-1). As plaques grow larger, they reduce the flow of blood through the arteries.

When blood flow to the heart muscle is restricted, chest pain *(angina pectoris)* may result, particularly during strenuous activity. This is the heart's way of saying it isn't getting enough oxygen. Angina often subsides when you rest, since a resting heart doesn't need as much oxygen as a working heart.

A *heart attack* occurs when blood flow through a coronary artery becomes completely blocked, either by progressive narrowing (stenosis) of a coronary artery, by the formation of a blood clot (thrombosis) in a coronary artery and/or spasm of the coronary arteries. With no oxygen and nutrients, the heart tissue supplied by the blocked artery begins to die. (Narrowing of the arteries that supply the brain with blood can increase the risk of stroke, too. A stroke occurs when the blood supply to the brain is interrupted, either by a blood clot that lodges in a blood vessel, or by bleeding from a broken blood vessel.)

Atherosclerosis doesn't just happen overnight—or immediately after menopause, for that matter. Rather, it's a gradual process that takes years—possibly half a lifetime or more—to develop. Researchers studying the risk of heart disease among children in the town of Bogalusa, Louisiana, found that *children as young as age ten have fatty streaks in their arteries that are believed to develop later into artery-clogging plaques.*

Certain risk factors may increase your chances of developing coronary heart disease. You're considered to be at a greater risk of developing coronary heart disease if you

- are over age fifty
- have high cholesterol
- have high blood pressure
- smoke cigarettes
- don't exercise
- are overweight
- have diabetes

How Estrogen Protects Against Heart Disease

Men are more vulnerable to heart disease than women—at least until menopause. The fact that women are relatively immune from heart disease until menopause, when estrogen levels fall, has led to the belief that estrogen somehow *protects* women from coronary heart disease. The theory has been bolstered in the last ten years or so by numerous studies showing that estrogen does indeed protect postmenopausal women against heart disease. Collectively, the studies have shown that *postmenopausal women who take oral estrogens for ten years or more have 50 percent less coronary heart disease than postmenopausal women who don't take hor-*

mones. Apparently, estrogen protects in a variety of different ways.

Estrogen and Cholesterol

As we mentioned earlier, cholesterol, a fatty substance that circulates in the bloodstream, is a major contributor to coronary heart disease. The development of plaques is strongly associated with high levels of cholesterol circulating in the bloodstream. As it turns out, estrogen has a powerful effect on blood lipids (fats) and cholesterol. Our studies and those of other researchers have shown that blood cholesterol levels rise sharply after menopause—an average of twenty-five points. This translates into roughly a 50 percent increase in your risk of developing heart disease.

But estrogen's effects on *total* cholesterol are only part of the story. Estrogen also has been found to *lower* levels of *low-density lipoproteins*, or LDL cholesterol. This is the "bad" cholesterol that builds up on and narrows the artery walls. Postmenopausal women who take oral estrogen also experience a rise in *high-density lipoproteins*, or HDL cholesterol, the "good" cholesterol that helps clear LDL cholesterol from the bloodstream. The percentage change in blood lipids depends on the amount of estrogen you take: the higher the dosage, the greater the change. On average, women who take a higher dosage of oral conjugated estrogen—1.25 mg per day—experience a rise in HDL cholesterol of 14 to 17 percent, while LDL cholesterol falls an average of 8 percent. In our 1990 study investigating the effects of oral estrogen on blood lipids, women taking 1.25 mg of estrogen (estropipate) daily experienced an increase of nearly 10 percent in HDL cholesterol after twelve months, a drop of 8 percent in LDL cholesterol, and a marked improvement in the ratios of total cholesterol to HDL cholesterol, all of which help protect against heart disease.

Estrogen and Blood Pressure

Elevated blood pressure is one of the most powerful contributors to coronary heart disease. Even mild elevations in blood pressure can lead to a greater incidence of premature atherosclerosis, heart attacks, and strokes. Clearly, a major goal of preventing a heart attack is to keep blood pressure in check. Since the older birth control pills containing high levels of synthetic estrogen and progestogens were known to raise blood pressure among a small percentage of women who took them, it was feared that postmenopausal estrogen might have the same effect on blood pressure. Contrary to popular belief, however, postmenopausal estrogen *doesn't* raise blood pressure. In fact, several studies have found that oral estrogen can actually *decrease* blood pressure. In a 1990 study we conducted, women who took estrogen alone experienced an average 3.8 percent decrease in blood pressure, and an even greater decrease in blood pressure when they took estrogen and exercised regularly.

Estrogen and Blood Clots

Blood clots play such a critical role in triggering a heart attack or stroke that the condition might be more appropriately named *atherothrombosis* (a *thrombosis* is a blood clot that lodges in a major artery). When a blood clot forms in a vital artery, it can trigger a life-threatening heart attack or stroke.

The sophisticated system of chemical checks and balances that controls blood clots and bleeding in the body is known as *hemostasis*. Hemostasis is a complex process, involving the blood vessel itself, specialized cells that circulate in the bloodstream, known as *platelets*, and dozens of *coagulation factors* and *anticoagulation factors* in the blood.

Oral estrogen has come under suspicion for increasing the risk of blood clots because it is known to increase the liver's production of several different coagulation factors. However, these coagulation factors are not biologically active until they're exposed to an injured blood vessel. Plus, "normal" levels of many of these coagulation factors vary widely, and it's impossible to predict who is at higher risk of developing blood clots by measuring levels of these enzymes.

On the other hand, our studies have found that estrogen *doesn't have any effect at all* on anticoagulants, particularly antithrombin III, which is a good marker for predicting whether you will develop a blood clot. In addition, we've found that menopause itself raises levels of potential anticlotting factors, such as *plasminogen*, possibly providing some natural protection against the formation of blood clots. This may help explain why postmenopausal estrogen therapy appears less likely to cause blood clots in older women. In fact, *there is no study showing a cause-and-effect relationship between taking estrogen and the development of blood clots*. Estrogen's poor reputation comes from studies on the use of older, high-dose oral contraceptives among older women who smoked. *Smoking is the demon!*

Estrogen and Insulin

High levels of *insulin*, a hormone produced by the pancreas to help maintain blood-sugar levels, appear to stimulate the *sympathetic nervous system*, resulting in elevated blood pressure, a known risk factor for coronary heart disease. High blood-sugar levels are also believed to somehow damage or alter the lining of the artery walls, allowing insulin to interact with the underlying tissues and making them more sensitive to the development of artery-narrowing plaques. As a result, high insulin levels are associated with an increased risk of heart disease.

Estrogen *decreases* fasting blood-sugar levels, possibly because it prevents the breakdown of insulin and helps insulin function more efficiently. This may provide added protection against heart disease.

Other Ways That Estrogen Protects

Estrogen may protect in other ways, as well: For instance, estrogen improves blood flow. The hormone also appears to somehow protect the innermost lining of the blood vessel walls, where artery-narrowing plaques form. At least three studies have shown that women who take estrogen are less likely to have occluded arteries. Angiograms, in which a dye is injected into the bloodstream and an X ray is taken as the dye passes through the coronary arteries, have shown that estrogen users have significantly less stenosis (narrowing) than nonusers, even when other risk factors, including hypertension, diabetes, cigarette smoking and obesity, are taken into account. In addition, estrogen helps to prevent spasm of the coronary arteries which can also trigger a heart attack. Indeed, estrogen appears to reduce the risk of severe coronary artery disease by a striking 56 to 63 percent.

What About Progestegen?

The picture grows a little more complicated when progestogen (a synthetic form of the reproductive hormone progesterone) is added. You may have heard reports that progestogen, which is often prescribed along with estrogen to protect against endometrial cancer, may cancel out estrogen's protective effect, and may possibly even *raise* your risk of heart disease. Long-term studies are now underway to determine the exact role of postmenopausal progestogen in the development of heart disease. However, preliminary results suggest the fear of heart disease associated with progestogen use may be exaggerated. A 1988 study of the use of combination oral contraceptives (containing estrogen and progestogen) among more than 100,000 women by Meir Stampfer, M.D., and colleagues at Harvard Medical School in Boston found no increased risk of cardiovascular disease among women who had used oral contraceptives in the past. In fact, the relative risk of major coronary disease for users was 20 percent *lower* than the risk for nonusers.

Progestogens *do* appear to somewhat dampen the effects of estrogen on blood lipids. However, the cyclic use of progestogens with intermediate doses of oral estrogen (.625 mg per day of Premarin or the equivalent) still results in a meaningful *overall increase in cardioprotective factors*, such as an increase in HDL cholesterol. For instance, one study showed that the combination of a progestogen and oral estrogen lowered LDL cholesterol and raised protective HDL cholesterol. Although the increase in HDL—6 percent—was about half that of women receiving estrogen alone, it was still substantial enough to confer added protection against heart disease.

In the near future, new types of progestogens and different ways of administering the hormone may make the whole issue of progestogen's effects on blood lipids obsolete. Preliminary evidence suggests that new types of synthetic progestogens, called *gestodene*, *desogestrel*, and *norgestimate* as well as oral micronized progesterone, will have little effect on HDL cholesterol in women taking estrogen. A transdermal skin patch containing both progestogen and estrogen may also reduce the negative effects of progestogen on blood lipids because the skin patch allows the hormones to enter the bloodstream without first passing through the liver.

Contrary to popular belief, the low levels of progestogen used in today's oral contraceptives have no adverse effect on blood pressure. Again, the idea that progestogens raise blood pressure was based on studies involving the older oral contraceptives, which contained large doses of progestogen.

As for blood clots, progestogen may even help protect against them. We found that postmenopausal progestogens *increase* the activity of the anticoagulant plasminogen from 16 to 20 percent. Although we don't yet know what effect these changes have in the body, it's possible that they have a protective effect. This effect of progestogens on plasminogen may be particularly important in the prevention of heart disease. It's possible that the higher levels of plasminogen among women taking progestogens may help guard against the ill effects of a protein carrier of cholesterol known as apolipoprotein (a) on the artery wall. Apolipoprotein (a) is genetically similar to plasminogen and high levels of apolipoprotein (a) may raise your risk of developing a blood clot.

Progestogens *do* increase insulin resistance somewhat, which may be a problem for some women, particularly those with diabetes. These women may need to be more closely monitored.

Animal studies have also suggested that progestogens may *reduce* blood flow, and this may dampen the positive effects that estrogen has on blood flow, particularly through the coronary arteries.

Overall, however, it appears that progestogens don't totally cancel out the good that estrogen does for your heart. In fact, progestogens may add some protective measures of their own!

Should You Take Hormone Additive Therapy to Protect Against Heart Disease?

Before deciding whether or not to take postmenopausal hormones to protect yourself against heart disease, you should have a complete physical examination and a *lipid profile* (a fasting blood test that measures total cholesterol, LDL cholesterol, HDL cholesterol, triglycerides, and the ratio of total to HDL cholesterol) to help gauge your risk of heart disease. (See "Cholesterol Tests: What the Results Mean," on page 67.) You should seriously consider taking hormone additive therapy if you

•have a family history of premature heart disease (a father or brother who develops heart disease before age fifty-five or a mother or sister who develops heart disease before age sixty)

•have high blood cholesterol levels (total cholesterol above 240 milligrams per deciliter of blood)

•have high blood pressure (diastolic pressure—the bottom number—above 95)

•have experienced a premature menopause (before age forty)

Cholesterol Tests: What the Results Mean

Total cholesterol
Below 200 mg/dl   Desirable
200 to 239 mg/dl   Borderline high risk
240 mg/dl or above   High risk

Low density lipoproteins
Below 130 mg/dl   Desirable
130 to 159 mg/dl   Borderline high risk
160 mg/dl or above   High risk

High density lipoproteins
Below 35 mg/dl   Increased risk
35 to 50 mg/dl   Good
50 mg/dl or above   Better

Triglycerides
20 to 140 mg/dl   Normal
140 to 190 mg/dl   Above normal—monitor
Above 190 mg/dl   High

Total cholesterol/HDL cholesterol
Above 4.4   Increased risk
Below 4.4   Desirable

Preventing Heart Disease: What You Can Do
Whether or not you take estrogen, your program of prevention should also include the following measures:

1. *Follow a low-fat, low-cholesterol diet.* Use our Prudent Diet for Heart Disease Prevention, outlined here, as a guide.

•Reduce the amount of total and saturated fat and cholesterol in your diet. Meat and dairy products are the main sources of fat in the typical American diet, and cutting back on these foods is an ideal place to start. A few tips: eat smaller portions of meat (two three-ounce servings per day, along with protein from milk, will suffice); choose leaner meats, such as fish, poultry with the skin removed, veal, and beef round and sirloin; trim the visible fat from meat before cooking; cook with the least amount of fat (broiling, braising, and stewing are best); and choose low-fat and no-fat milk and dairy products.

•Eat foods high in soluble fiber (up to 35 grams) every day. Soluble fiber, one of two types of dietary fiber, helps lower LDL cholesterol. Foods high in soluble fiber include dried peas and beans and, yes, even oat bran.

•Eat foods high in beta carotene and other antioxidants. Yellow and orange fruits and vegetables are chock full of these nutrients, which may protect against damage to LDL cholesterol from oxygen free radicals. Oxidation of LDL cholesterol by free radicals is now believed to make it more likely to develop into artery-clogging plaques.

•Drink coffee in moderation (no more than three cups per day)—particularly *decaffeinated* coffee. There's no evidence to date that regular coffee contributes to heart disease, and only sketchy evidence that de-caffeinated coffee does. But there's also no good reason to drink a lot of coffee.

•Limit the amount of sodium in your diet to about one teaspoon (2,000 milligrams) per day to help control your blood pressure.

•Eat plenty of calcium-rich foods (milk, cottage cheese, yogurt, collards, bok choy, Kale, and broccoli). A high-calcium diet (1,500 milligrams per day) may help prevent hypertension. (For a list of foods high in calcium, see page 147.)

•Eat fish at least twice a week. Fish and fish oils may help protect against blood clots.

•Drink alcohol only in moderation (no more than two drinks per day).

•Eat several small meals throughout the day instead of three large meals. People who do so have lower cho-lesterol levels.

•Consume the majority of your calories before 5:00 P.M., when they're more likely to be used for en-ergy than stored as fat—and possibly as cholesterol de-posits in your arteries.

2. *Quit smoking.* Nearly three times more smokers die of heart disease than lung cancer. Carbon monoxide in cigarette smoke reduces the blood's oxygen-carrying ability, so there's less oxygen available to your heart and other organs. Cigarette smoking raises levels of LDL cholesterol, decreases HDL cholesterol, and dam-ages the lining of the coronary arteries, setting the stage for the development of coronary lesions. Cigarette smoking also adversely affects blood coagulation, which may encourage the development of blood clots in smokers.

No matter how long you've smoked, when you quit

your risk of heart disease begins to decline. *Within two years of quitting, your chances of having a heart attack will be cut in half. Ten years after quitting, your risk of dying from a heart attack will be almost the same as if you'd never smoked.* So do your heart a big favor and quit.

3. *Exercise.* Sedentary living is now considered a major risk factor for heart disease, along with high blood pressure, high blood cholesterol, and cigarette smoking. Conversely, regular physical activity appears to be a powerful deterrent against heart disease. Exercise lowers your blood pressure and heart rate; burns body fat, which helps counter obesity, a serious risk factor for heart disease; promotes more efficient use of insulin by your body, which may reduce your risk of developing adult-onset diabetes; raises levels of protective HDL cholesterol and lowers LDL cholesterol; may even help prevent blood clots; and reduces stress, which may contribute to an increased risk of heart disease.

For protection against heart disease, *any* kind of physical activity is better than none. However, some activities are clearly better than others. We recommend aerobic activities—those that involve increasing your heart rate and breathing and using the large muscles of your body—for twenty minutes three times a week or preferably thirty minutes five times per week. Brisk walking, bicycling, and swimming are ideal for women in midlife.

4. *Drink alcohol in moderation.* There's some evidence that alcohol may help prevent heart disease—but *only* in moderate amounts (no more than one or two drinks per day). Alcohol appears to protect against coronary heart disease by raising levels of HDL cholesterol. Moderate alcohol consumption is also associated with several favorable changes in blood coagulation, which could also explain its possible protective effect. Alcohol apparently decreases the "stickiness" of blood platelets, and increases the anticoagulant prostacyclin. Alcohol also interacts with aspirin to prolong the time blood takes to clot (It's not a good idea to take aspirin and drink alcohol at the same time, however; doing so may accelerate the rate at which alcohol enters your blood stream). Finally, alcohol lowers the level of fibrinogen, a potent risk factor for coronary heart disease. On the other hand, studies have also found moderate drinkers to be at a higher risk of suffering a cerebral hemorrhage, a type of stroke caused by bleeding from a broken blood vessel. *Heavy drinking* (more than three drinks per day) can actually do more harm than good, damaging the heart muscle, triggering disturbances in the heart's rhythm, reducing blood flow from the heart, raising blood triglyceride levels (a possible risk factor for women), and raising blood pressure. So more isn't better.

5. *Keep your blood pressure in check.* The higher your blood pressure, the greater is the risk of suffering a heart attack or stroke. For every five to six points your blood pressure is reduced, the risk of heart disease declines by 20 to 25 percent, and the risk of stroke by 30 to 40 percent. Exercise, eating a low-sodium diet, and keeping your weight in check are ideal ways to lower your blood pressure. Your physician can prescribe blood pressure lowering medications if life-style measures fail to do the trick.

6. *Control your weight.* Studies have found that even mildly overweight women are up to forty times more likely to develop coronary heart disease than normal weight women. Women who gain weight *during the*

middle years have double the risk of developing coronary heart disease of women who have been overweight all their lives. Women who tend to put on weight around the waist and abdomen ("apple" shapes) are more likely to have lower levels of HDL cholesterol, elevated LDL cholesterol, triglycerides and insulin, and are more likely to develop hypertension and adult-onset diabetes. Losing weight is often enough to lower elevated blood cholesterol and blood pressure, and to keep adult-onset diabetes in check without drugs and their sometimes serious side effects.

If you have a weight problem, simply cutting back on fat in your diet and increasing your physical activity may solve it. If these measures don't work, ask your doctor for help, or check out some of the more reputable organized weight loss programs, such as Weight Watchers or the TOPS Club (Taking Off Pounds Sensibly). Check the phone book for a local affiliate.

7. *Keep tabs on diabetes.* Diabetes mellitus is particularly hard on women. Several studies have confirmed that the condition somehow completely wipes out the biological protection against heart disease that healthy women enjoy. Heart disease is just one of several major complications associated with diabetes, including kidney failure, amputations due to infection, and blindness. Better control of diabetes is associated with fewer complications. And the majority of women with adult-onset diabetes can control it with dietary changes alone. But don't attempt to treat this serious metabolic disorder by yourself. Rather, plan to work closely with your physician (and possibly a registered dietitian), who will develop an eating plan to control your diabetes and prescribe blood-sugar lowering medications, if necessary.

8. *Ask your physician about taking aspirin.* When you take aspirin regularly, your blood becomes more resistant to forming a clot. But before you begin taking aspirin, first discuss it with your doctor. Although aspirin is readily available over the counter, it's not safe for everybody. If you have liver or kidney disease, a peptic ulcer, gastrointestinal bleeding or other bleeding problems, you may not be able to take aspirin at all, or you may need to adjust the amount you take. Since aspirin prolongs bleeding, you should notify your physician that you're taking aspirin if you're scheduled for any kind of surgery. Also, if you have uncontrolled hypertension or any condition that might increase the risk of a cerebral hemorrhage (a type of stroke caused by bleeding from a broken blood vessel in the brain), you should not take aspirin routinely without first checking with your physician. When we prescribe aspirin to patients in our clinic, we recommend taking a junior aspirin (60 milligrams) every three days, which seems sufficient in most cases.

9. *Control stress.* Events you find emotionally taxing—getting stuck in a traffic jam on the way to the airport, for example—can trigger a physiological response in the body called the "fight or flight response," in which your body releases a flood of chemicals from the adrenal glands, notably *epinephrine* and *norepinephrine*. These hormones accelerate your breathing and heart rate, raise your blood pressure and blood-sugar levels, and release high-energy fats into the bloodstream for quick energy—essentially preparing you for a fight with or a quick flight away from a physical threat. The hormones also increase the stickiness of blood platelets, which make blood clot more easily (in case you're wounded in the ensuing battle). *Cortisol*, another hormone released from the adrenal glands when your body is chronically stressed, raises blood cholesterol levels.

Several studies have suggested that the constant firing of the fight or flight response from living in a stressful world may lead to permanent increases in heart rate and blood pressure. Blood cholesterol levels may also be grossly elevated by chronic stress.

Although many questions remain unanswered about the role of stress and heart disease, it makes sense to take stock of the stresses in your life, and reduce stress whenever possible. Exercising regularly is an ideal place to start, since it also helps protect against heart disease and high blood pressure. Relaxation techniques, such as deep breathing, progressive muscular relaxation, yoga, meditation, and biofeedback can also help undo the effects of stress on your body. Preliminary studies suggest that long-term use of these procedures may *permanently* decrease your body's response to the stress hormone norepinephrine.

10. *See your doctor regularly.* Regular medical checkups can help monitor your condition—and tell you how effective your efforts are. If diet, exercise, and other life-style changes or hormone additive therapy aren't effective in lowering your cholesterol, your physician may prescribe certain cholesterol-lowering drugs, including *cholestyramine* (Cholybar, Questran), *colestipol* (Colestid, Cholestabyl), a prescription form of the B-vitamin *niacin, lovastatin,* (Mevacor), *simvastatin* (Zocor), *gemfibrozil* (Lopid), or *psyllium seed,* found in over-the-counter bulk fiber laxatives, such as Metamucil.

CHAPTER 6

❧

Estrogen and Your Bones

We all lose bone mass as we age. After menopause, the gradual loss of bone mass associated with normal aging occurs at a more rapid rate—primarily because of the drop in estrogen at this time in a woman's life. If you have low bone mass before menopause or if you rapidly lose bone mass for many years after menopause, your bones may weaken to the point that debilitating fractures occur with even the slightest provocation—a condition known as *osteoporosis*. Osteoporosis is a crippling, painful condition affecting one out of every four postmenopausal women. It is the twelfth leading cause of death among women today. The cost to individuals and society is enormous: about $10 billion is spent each year on acute care associated with fractures resulting from osteoporosis. This does not include hired nursing care, nursing home stays, or costs attributable to changes in life-style as a result of disability from a fracture.

Fortunately, osteoporosis can be prevented. And a key to prevention for some women is judicious use of hormone additive therapy.

What Is Osteoporosis?

In simplest terms, osteoporosis is a condition marked by severe or prolonged bone loss that makes bones less likely to withstand the physical stresses of everyday living. Just how this bone loss occurs is more complicated. To understand the process, you'll need to know a few basics about your bones.

Although you probably don't think much about them, the 206 bones in your body play a vital role in your health and well-being. Your bones give you support, allow you to go about your daily activities, and protect your vital organs. Bone marrow manufactures new blood cells. Your bones are a virtual warehouse for storing calcium, a mineral needed for muscle contraction, blood clotting, and nerve impulse transmission. In fact, 99 percent of the calcium in your body is stored in your bones.

Each of the bones in your body is made up of two types of bone tissue: *trabecular bone* consists of a network of bony plates resembling latticework or scaffolding that is lightweight yet extremely strong. Trabecular bone is found mostly in the vertebrae of the spine, in the breastbone, in the top of the pelvis, and in the ends of the long bones of your body (arms and legs). Surrounding the trabecular bone is a thin sheet of denser *cortical bone*. Cortical bone is also the major type of bone tissue in the arms and legs.

Your bone mass—the total amount of bone in your skeleton—is maintained by a delicate balance between the breakdown of old bone and the formation of new bone, an ongoing process known as *bone remodeling*. Two major cells are involved in bone remodeling: *Osteoclasts* are responsible for removing old cells. Once activated, osteoclasts secrete powerful enzymes that dissolve old bone cells, carving out microscopic cavities in the bone. *Osteoblasts* are smaller cells that are somehow attracted to the hollowed out spaces made by osteoclasts. Osteoblasts manufacture the basic building material of bone, known as *osteoid*, or bone matrix, consisting mostly of collagen fibers. About ten days after the osteoid has been laid down, crystals—mostly of calcium and phosphorus—are added to the framework, a process called *bone mineralization*.

How Bone Loss Occurs

From the time you are born until you reach early adulthood, you produce more new bone tissue than you lose through bone breakdown. Around age thirty-five, however, you reach *peak bone mass* and an imbalance in the bone remodeling cycle develops, so that old bone removal outpaces new bone replacement. We're not sure why this is so. It may be that the chemical "switches" that normally signal osteoblasts to lay down new bone are no longer effective. Calcium absorption declines with age, too, partly because of a decrease in your body's manufacture of vitamin D, and partly because of the drop in estrogen after menopause (estrogen enhances the body's ability to absorb calcium). As a result of these changes, blood calcium levels decline. To bring blood calcium levels back to normal, the body signals the bones to release stored calcium into the bloodstream. Because of these changes, either osteoclasts carve out cavities that are too deep, or osteoblasts don't make enough new bone to fill existing cavities, and you lose bone mass.

From age thirty-five until menopause, you lose cortical bone at a rate of .3 to .5 percent per year. After menopause and until about age sixty-five, the rate of cortical bone loss increases to about 1 percent per year, slowing down after age sixty-five to 0.18 percent per year. Some experts believe you experience a steady loss of trabecular bone after you reach peak bone mass in your twenties. Others say the bone loss pattern for trabecular bone is similar to that for cortical bone; that is, you lose 0.19 percent per year before menopause, increasing to 1.1 percent thereafter.

The bottom line is that a woman can expect to lose about 35 percent of her cortical bone and 50 percent of her trabecular bone over a lifetime. Men lose only about two-thirds these amounts.

The End Result of Osteoporosis: Fractures

Under severe stress or trauma, *any* bone can break. However, bones weakened by progressive loss of bone mass will break more easily. The most vulnerable bones are the vertebrae of the spine, which are composed primarily of latticelike trabecular bone. As the vertebrae become more porous and weak over the years, they go through various stages of structural deformity and can actually collapse. Unlike fractures of other bones in the body, which can mend themselves under the proper conditions, the structural damage to the spinal vertebrae cannot be undone.

Hip fractures (actually, fractures of the upper part of the thigh bone, or *femur*)—usually the result of an accident or injury—are by far the most disabling and life-threatening consequence of osteoporosis. *Fewer than one-half of all women who suffer a hip fracture regain normal function. Fifteen percent of women die shortly after their injury, and nearly 30 percent die within one year.* Deaths from hip fractures are not caused by the fracture itself, but from some condition resulting from confinement to a hospital or nursing home bed, such as pneumonia, thrombosis (blood clots), or a fat embolism (bone marrow fat trapped in the lung). So you can see why preventing the bone loss that can lead to fractures is imperative.

How Estrogen Protects Your Bones

A number of factors contribute to the development of osteoporosis: adequate calcium intake over the course of a lifetime; regular exercise, which helps build bone mass; whether or not you smoke cigarettes, which lowers estrogen levels in the body; how much alcohol you drink; and whether you have a family history of osteoporosis. One of the most important factors at the time of menopause (or surgical menopause) is low estrogen levels, which accelerate the rate of bone loss. For this reason, estrogen therapy is one of the most effective means we have of slowing or even stopping the accelerated loss of bone mass after menopause.

Estrogen is believed to help slow bone loss in several ways:

•Estrogen somehow preserves bone mineral, which in turn is associated with a decrease in fractures among women who take it. Estrogen receptors have been found in osteoblasts, the cells responsible for laying down new bone, suggesting that estrogen has a direct effect on bone.

•Estrogen also interacts with several other "bone hormones," and in this way indirectly influences the regulation of bone mass. Estrogen blocks the bone-dissolving actions of parathyroid hormone. It stimulates the activation of vitamin D, which increases the absorp-

tion of calcium in the intestines and increases the reab-
sorption of calcium through the kidneys. Estrogen also
stimulates *calcitonin*, a bone-sparing hormone released
by the thyroid gland and other tissues. Calcitonin slows
the breakdown of old bone by osteoclasts. Finally, estrogen stimulates the liver to produce proteins that bind
to certain hormones released from the adrenal glands,
decreasing their ability to dissolve bone.

•Estrogen increases your body's ability to absorb calcium from the intestines. Your bones need calcium for
mineralization, the process by which newly formed
bone becomes hard. Some studies have even suggested
that because they are more efficient at absorbing calcium, women on estrogen therapy can get by with a
daily requirement of 1,200 mg of calcium, rather than
the recommended 1,500 mg per day for postmenopausal
women.

•Estrogen increases collagen in other parts of the
body (notably the skin), and we suspect that it does the
same in bone. Collagen in bone forms the bone matrix
to which calcium and phosphorous crystals adhere, giving bone its rigidity.

Estrogen may have an indirect effect, as well: By im-
proving your sense of well-being, it may increase your
level of activity. More active women are stronger and
more stable than sedentary women, which in turn, decreases their chances of falling.

Whatever the mechanism of action, estrogen prevents
loss of bone mass and considerably reduces your risk of
suffering a fracture. Bruce Ettinger, M.D., of Kaiser
Permanente in San Francisco, has determined that the
"bone mineral age" of women taking estrogen is ten to
twelve years less than their actual age.

Several long-term studies have shown that the use of estrogen is associated with a *dramatic* decline in fractures of the hip. The actual figures vary from study to study, but the average is about 50 percent. As for fractures of the spine, Robert Lindsay, M.D., of Columbia University in New York has shown a *90 percent decrease in spinal deformities* (such as loss of height and Dowager's hump) among surgically menopausal women who took estrogens for ten years. In his study, only 4 percent of women taking estrogen suffered spinal vertebral fractures, compared to 38 percent of untreated women.

What About Progestogen?

The hormone progesterone appears to help protect bone mass, too. Low levels of progesterone have been associated with loss of bone mass in premenopausal women whose estrogen levels are normal. Progesterone is thought to prevent the bone-dissolving adrenal hormones from attaching to bone cell receptors, thus offering further protection to bone.

Several studies have suggested that progestogen may even help promote the formation of new bone when given together with estrogen. In a ten-year study by Lila Nachtigall, M.D., and colleagues at New York University Medical Center, women who started taking combination estrogen/progestogen therapy within three years after their final menstrual period actually experienced an *increase* in bone density. Women who started therapy more than three years after menopause experienced some loss of bone density, but not as much as the women who took no hormones whatsoever. Yet another study by Claus Christiansen, M.D., and colleagues at the University of Copenhagen in Denmark, found that bone density *increased* during the three years that study participants took a combination of estrogen and progestogen.

Although progestogens given by themselves aren't as good as a combination of estrogen and progestogen, they do work. One type of progestogen, *megestrol acetate* (Megace), is useful for protecting bone in women who've had breast cancer and can't take estrogen therapy.

Estrogen and progestogen help protect bone in different ways and, therefore, taking a combination of estrogen and progestogen provides added protection. This is one reason why women who have had a hysterectomy and who have lost more than 30 percent of peak bone mass may want to consider taking combination therapy, even though progestogen is not needed to protect the endometrial lining.

Should You Take Estrogen to Prevent Osteoporosis?

Some women are more likely than others to develop osteoporosis, and these women should consider taking estrogen to prevent osteoporosis. Characteristically, women at risk are described as white (Caucasian) or Asian, blond, petite, with a small body frame, or with a family history of osteoporosis. Women are especially at risk if they have had a premature or surgical menopause and have not taken postmenopausal hormone therapy.

You should know, however, that while these risk factors can give you and your physician an idea of whether you will later develop osteoporosis, their powers of prediction are limited. By some estimates, using risk factors to determine who will develop osteoporosis detects only 30 percent of all women actually at risk.

A much more effective way of determining whether you are at risk and need estrogen is to have your bone density tested. Bone density testing is the only definitive way to determine how much bone density you have now, and what effect your menopause is having on your bone density. There are several methods now available for determining bone density, but one of the quickest, safest, and most reliable screening tests for osteoporosis involves having a portion of your wrist scanned with *dual energy X-ray absorptiometry* (DEXA). The test, which involves placing your wrist under a specialized x-ray scanner, takes just a few minutes to perform and exposes you to just a fraction of the X-ray radiation of an ordinary arm X-ray.

Another simple and reliable screening test is *radiographic densitometry*, in which your hand is placed alongside a standardized aluminum wedge and a routine X-ray is taken. The X-ray is then scanned by a computer and the bone density of your finger is compared with that of the aluminum wedge.

Yet another screening test involves the use of *single photon absorptiometry* (SPA) to measure the bone density of your wrist or heel.

If your bone density is found to be low during a screening with DEXA, radiographic densitometry, or SPA, additional tests may be necessary to determine the bone density of the more vulnerable "fracture zones," such as the hip and spine. Your physician also has several blood and urine tests that can help determine the rate at which you are losing bone, including a test that determines the ratio of *calcium-to-creatinine* in the urine and a test that measures levels of the enzyme *alkaline phosphatase* in the blood. Both tests can help determine the activity of the bone remodeling cycle (the breakdown of old bone and the formation of new bone). Ask your doctor about these and other tests.

The technology for bone density testing is fairly new and may not yet be available from your physician. If your doctor cannot provide a referral, contact the National Osteoporosis Foundation, 1150 17th Street, N.W., Suite 500, Washington, D.C. 20036, for a list of physicians, hospitals, and clinics near you that offer bone density testing.

Preventing Osteoporosis: What You Can Do
Again, taking estrogen is one way to stave off accelerated bone loss that can lead to osteoporosis. But it's not the only way. Even if you *do* take estrogen, you can enhance its effects by also incorporating the following life-style measures.

1. *Exercise regularly.* Exercise is the only preventive measure that not only halts bone loss but also *stimulates the formation of new bone*. Bone responds to physical stress in the same way muscles do: by becoming bigger and stronger. Generally speaking, weight-bearing or load-bearing activities—that is, exercises that put stress on the long bones of the body, such as walking, stair climbing, stair-stepping, aerobic dance, and bicycling—are best for building bone mass and slowing bone loss.

But don't overdo it. Repeated and prolonged exercise (marathon running, for example) can cause bone fatigue

and microscopic fractures. And exercise-induced amen-
orrhea (cessation of menstruation caused by strenuous
exercise over a matter of months or years) in your premenopausal years can actually cause you to *lose* trabecular bone in the spine. The bone loss is believed to be
caused by a drop in estrogen associated with decreased
body fat, and may be permanent.

2. *Eat a diet adequate in calcium.* If you don't get
enough calcium in your diet throughout your life, your
bones will suffer. This is because bone is roughly two-
thirds mineral by weight, and calcium makes up about
40 percent of that mineral. In a classic study comparing
bone mass in two groups from different rural areas in
Yugoslavia—one group having an average daily calcium intake (940 milligrams) that was twice that of the
other (441 milligrams), women in the higher-calcium
group definitely had stronger bones at skeletal maturity
and a lower incidence of hip fractures later in life than
women in the low-calcium group.

Generally speaking, the *source* of calcium in your
diet—whether it be from food or supplements—isn't all
that essential. The important thing is *to take in enough
calcium on a regular basis to create a positive calcium
balance*, in which you consume more calcium than your
body excretes through urine, feces, and sweat. Low-fat
dairy products, such as skim milk, low-fat yogurt, and
nonfat dry milk, are excellent sources of calcium.
Green leafy vegetables (except spinach, whose calcium
is bound up and not very available), shellfish, almonds,
Brazil nuts, tofu, and small fish (such as sardines with
their bones) are high in calcium, too. Fortified foods,
including orange juice (Minute Maid), calcium-fortified
specialty breads, and even calcium-fortified milk
(Calcimilk), are good sources, as well. (To find out if

you're getting enough calcium in your diet, fill out our Calcium Questionnaire on page 147 of the appendix.)

3. *Take a calcium supplement.* It's almost impossible to get the amount of calcium you need from food alone, and calcium supplements provide an excellent, calorie-free way to close the gap between your calcium intake from foods and the daily amount you need to stay in positive calcium balance. When choosing a supplement, only the *elemental* calcium is available for absorption. Calcium carbonate, the cheapest and most widely used ingredient in calcium supplements, contains the highest amount of calcium per tablet (40 percent of elemental calcium). Calcium citrate is the best absorbed of the most common types of supplemental calcium, but contains slightly less calcium per tablet. (You'll find many more tips on getting enough calcium from food and choosing the best supplements in our book, *Menopause and Midlife Health*).

4. *Watch out for "calcium robbers" in your diet.* These are foods and substances that hinder calcium absorption or cause your body to excrete it, including too much *dietary fiber* (more than 35 grams per day), *protein*, *sodium*, *caffeine*, and possibly *phosphorus* (found in soft drinks and certain other foods.)

5. *Get plenty of vitamin D.* Vitamin D helps to maintain a positive calcium balance. One recent study of a group of postmenopausal women in Boston showed that one-half of them became vitamin D deficient during the winter months, when exposure to sunlight was limited. Moreover, women whose daily vitamin D intake was below 220 international units (IU) had higher levels of bone-dissolving parathyroid hormone in their blood in the spring.

The recommended daily allowance for adults is 400

IU, which may be obtained either from your diet or from the sun. While the sun is your primary source of vitamin D, there is no way to measure how much you are getting. Some experts estimate that a white woman needs from fifteen minutes to one hour of sunshine daily to meet her vitamin D requirement. (Keep in mind that regular use of a sunscreen may limit vitamin D production in your skin.) Vitamin D in the diet is fairly limited: fatty fish, butter, eggs, liver, and fortified milk are the best sources. Most multivitamin preparations also contain the 400 units you need each day. But don't overdo it; too much vitamin D can stimulate bone loss. Avoid amounts in excess of 1,000 units per day.

6. *Don't smoke.* Several studies have associated cigarette smoking with an accelerated loss of bone and a greater risk of osteoporosis. Cigarette smoking changes the liver's metabolism of estrogen, making it less biologically active. Cigarette smokers also experience menopause an average of two to three years earlier than nonsmokers, meaning that smokers experience the accelerated rate of bone loss associated with menopause that much earlier than nonsmokers. Too, there's some evidence that cigarette smoking somehow inhibits new bone cell formation.

7. *Drink alcohol only in moderation.* Alcoholics have a lower bone mass than nondrinkers. However, having as few as three drinks per day on a regular basis may contribute to low bone mass. Excessive alcohol consumption is typically associated with poor nutrition, including low intakes of calcium and vitamin D. Alcohol also appears to impair the liver's ability to activate vitamin D. Alcohol inhibits calcium absorption, too. Until we know more about the effects of alcohol on bone mass, limit your alcohol consumption to no more than two drinks per day.

8. *Avoid medications that interfere with calcium absorption.* Aluminum in some antacids binds to and lowers levels of phosphorus which, in turn, increases calcium excretion. If your antacid contains aluminum, consider switching to a brand that doesn't.

Antacids containing aluminum: AlternaGEL liquid, Amphojel, Basaljel, Maalox, Mylanta, Nephrox, Rolaids, WinGel.

Antacids without aluminum: Alka-Seltzer, baking soda, Citrocarbonate antacid, Milk of Magnesia, Riopan, Tums.

Other medications that cause you to excrete more calcium are *steroids* (often prescribed to reduce the inflammation of asthma, arthritis, and other inflammatory conditions), certain *diuretics* (in particular, *furosemide*, prescribed to relieve water retention associated with congestive heart failure, kidney disease, and cirrhosis of the liver), the antibiotic *tetracycline*, and long-term use of the antituberculosis drug, *isoniazid*. If you are taking any of these medications, you may want to discuss with your doctor alternative types of medications that don't promote bone loss.

If you already have osteoporosis, your doctor has a number of medications besides estrogen that can help protect you from further bone loss, height loss, and fractures. These include a prescription form of the hormone *calcitonin* (Calcimar, Miacalcin, Cibacalcin), substances known as *bisphosphonates* (Didronel), a prescription form of *vitamin D*, and *sodium fluoride*— the only drug that can actually help *build* new bone. (Although the use of sodium fluoride is still controversial, our clinical experience has shown that sodium fluoride works best when used in conjunction with estrogen.) Other potentially helpful drugs that have been associated with a decreased incidence of fractures or an increase in bone mass are *thiazide diuretics*, commonly used to treat hypertension.

CHAPTER 7

❀

The Risks of Hormone Therapy

You may have read or heard that estrogen therapy increases your risk of endometrial cancer and possibly breast cancer. Over the past several years, headlines like these spread a wave of fear over women taking estrogen—or those who were thinking about taking it. Let's look at the facts about these and other possible risks of hormone therapy to help ease some of your greatest fears.

Endometrial Cancer

Endometrial cancer, cancer of the lining of the uterus (not the uterus itself), is the most common cancer of the reproductive tract in the United States, affecting about one in one thousand women. But when caught in the precancerous stages, it can be treated without radical surgery, and the cure rate is virtually 100 percent.

You've probably heard that postmenopausal estrogens increase your risk of developing endometrial cancer. In fact, studies have shown that postmenopausal women who have not had a hysterectomy and who take estrogen without progestogen are from two to thirteen times more likely to develop endometrial cancer as nonusers. While the risk may sound high, it must be put into perspective. Essentially, ten to twenty out of every one thousand women who take estrogen alone will develop endometrial cancer, compared with one in one thousand nonusers. In fact, *more than 99 percent of postmenopausal estrogen users do not develop endometrial cancer*.

Moreover, most endometrial cancers associated with estrogen use are less aggressive and are usually caught earlier than those that develop among nonusers, so women with this type of endometrial cancer tend to have a good prognosis.

Since the first reports of an increased risk of endometrial cancer associated with the use of estrogen came out, physicians have begun prescribing progestogen along with estrogen for at least ten days per cycle. This regimen more closely resembles a woman's natural menstrual cycle and prevents overstimulation of the uterine lining by estrogen alone. As a result, the incidence of endometrial cancer among women taking combination hormone therapy *is less than that of women who take no hormones whatsoever*.

Remember, too, that estrogen alone increases the risk of endometrial cancer *only among postmenopausal women who still have an intact uterus*. If you have had a hysterectomy, you don't need to worry about taking estrogen alone, since you don't have a uterus. (During the recent scare about a link between estrogen and endometrial cancer, many women who had had a hysterectomy and didn't need to worry stopped treatment.)

Besides taking a progestogen along with estrogen if you have an intact uterus, there are a few other ways that you can protect yourself from endometrial cancer.

1. *If you are overweight, lose weight.* Women who are twenty-one to fifty pounds overweight are three times more likely to develop endometrial cancer than normal weight women; women weighing more than fifty pounds over their ideal weight have a nine-fold increased risk. Overweight women with a family history of endometrial, breast, or ovarian cancer are at a particularly greater risk.

2. *Take the progestogen challenge test.* Some physicians recommend that all postmenopausal women who have not had a hysterectomy and who are *not* taking hormone additive therapy undergo a test called the *progestogen challenge* once a year as a screening test for early stages of endometrial cancer. The test involves taking a progestogen every day for ten to thirteen days. If you experience *no bleeding*, the test is negative and should be repeated annually, providing you are not using hormones and remain symptom-free (that is, you experience no abnormal menstrual bleeding during the year). If you experience "withdrawal bleeding" after taking a progestogen, this is a sign that your uterine lining is being stimulated by estrogen and that you may be at an increased risk of developing endometrial cancer. Your physician may then recommend that you continue taking a progestogen for thirteen days each month for as long as withdrawal bleeding follows. Treatment of high risk women with progestogen usually eliminates their risk of developing this cancer altogether.

3. *Periodically undergo endometrial sampling.* This is a simple and fairly painless procedure that involves removing a sample of endometrial tissue from your uterus so it can be examined under a microscope for possible signs of cancer. The procedure can be performed—usually without anesthesia—right in your doctor's office. First, your doctor will perform a pelvic exam to evaluate the size and position of your uterus. After applying an antiseptic to the cervix and upper vagina, your doctor will insert a long, narrow plastic or metal suctioning device through the cervix into the uterus, where a sample of endometrial cells is obtained.

Because endometrial sampling is associated with some cramping and discomfort, you may want to take aspirin or ibuprofen (Advil, Nuprin, Motrin IB) an hour before the procedure. Sometimes, if your cervix has narrowed, or *stenosed*, your doctor may inject a local anesthetic into the cervix to ease discomfort.

Some physicians recommend a "baseline" evaluation of the endometrium before you begin taking hormone additive therapy. Others (ourselves included) prefer to wait until after you've taken hormones for three months.

4. *Have regular medical checkups while you are taking hormone additive therapy, and report any unusual bleeding patterns to your physician immediately.* The single most important early warning sign associated with endometrial cancer is abnormal uterine bleeding. Ninety percent of women with endometrial cancer will experience abnormal bleeding.

Of course, you can expect to experience some vaginal bleeding when you take hormone additive therapy. (How much and what kind of bleeding pattern you can expect are described on page 117.) If you take hormones, *any deviation from your normal bleeding pattern should be promptly reported to your doctor.*

Keep in mind, too, that not *all* abnormal bleeding is caused by endometrial cancer. Your physician has a number of diagnostic tests, such as endometrial sampling and ultrasound, that can be used to help determine the cause of the bleeding. And remember: The earlier the cancer is caught, the better is the prognosis.

Breast Cancer

This is the cancer women fear most, partly because it is the most common cancer among women (the incidence is rising; now one in nine women will develop breast cancer in her lifetime). Women also fear breast cancer because the scientific community doesn't know yet how to prevent it, and treatment often involves the loss of a breast, a prospect many women find more frightening than the cancer itself.

Because certain types of breast cancer are fueled by the hormone estrogen, and because a woman's age at menarche (start of menstruation), age at the birth of her first child, and age at menopause appear to affect her subsequent risk of developing breast cancer, postmenopausal hormones have come under scrutiny as a possible risk factor. Would the additional exposure to estrogen after menopause—when estrogen levels are normally low and when a woman's risk of cancer naturally rises with age—increase her chances of developing breast cancer?

The fear of breast cancer was fueled by a highly publicized Swedish study published in 1989 involving more than 23,000 women ages thirty-five and over. The researchers found that women using a combination of estrogen and progestogen experienced overall about 10 percent more breast cancers than expected—reflecting only a slightly elevated risk of breast cancer, which would be perfectly acceptable given the benefits associated with the use of postmenopausal estrogens. The researchers, however, also reported that among the 850 women in the study who took estrogen for nine years or more, the incidence of breast cancer increased to 70 percent above expected levels.

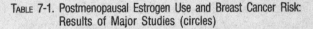

TABLE 7-1. Postmenopausal Estrogen Use and Breast Cancer Risk: Results of Major Studies (circles)

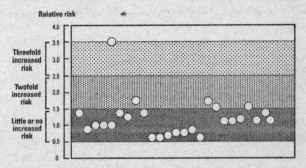

Chart adapted with permission from Dupont, W., Page D. L., "Menopausal Estrogen Replacement Therapy and Breast Cancer." *Archives of Internal Medicine*, Volume 151, January, 1991, pages 67–72.

More recently, however, a thorough analysis of the data—a *meta analysis* (a combination of all previous epidemiological studies)—shows that the risk of developing breast cancer is not all that great (see Table 7-1). After fifteen years of estrogen additive therapy, your risk of developing breast cancer may increase by roughly 30 percent, which is barely significant in statistical terms. No studies have shown an increase in deaths from breast cancer among estrogen users, and some have actually shown an increase in the cure rate of breast cancer among women taking postmenopausal hormones. It's not known whether the hormone therapy itself played a role in the higher cure rate or whether the women were screened more diligently, helping to catch their cancers in the early stages, when the cure rate is high.

The story is a little different if you have a family history of breast cancer, however. Studies have shown that among women with a family history of breast cancer, those who have ever used postmenopausal hormones have a twofold greater risk than those who have never taken them.

The exact mechanisms by which estrogen may increase the risk of breast cancer are not known. Estrogen doesn't appear to be an initiator of cancer; that is, it does not turn a normal cell into a cancerous cell. Rather estrogen appears to be a *promoter* of cancer by stimulating cells that have already become cancerous to grow more rapidly.

More research needs to be conducted before we fully understand the role of postmenopausal hormone therapy in the development of breast cancer. At this point, the benefits to some women (particularly those at risk of developing heart disease and osteoporosis) clearly outweigh the slightly increased risk of breast cancer. Remember: Ten times more women die of cardiovascular disease than of breast cancer.

Keep in mind, too, that postmenopausal hormone therapy isn't the only possible risk factor to consider: a high-fat diet may contribute to up to 30 percent of breast cancers, and reducing the fat in your diet certainly would be a prudent policy for lowering your risk of breast cancer. Based on the reports that have been conducted so far, the fat in your diet should be limited to *no more than 25 percent of your total daily calories*.

Being overweight in your postmenopausal years also raises your risk of breast cancer. This may be because excess body fat helps convert androgens produced by the adrenal glands in postmenopausal women into estrogen. Plus, overweight women have lower levels of a liver protein known as *sex hormone binding globulin*, which binds to estrogen in the bloodstream, making it less biologically active. The result: Heavier women have higher levels of more biologically active estrogen than women of normal weight.

Several studies have suggested that the amount of alcohol you drink may also affect your risk of breast cancer. The most convincing to date, a 1988 study conducted by Walter C. Willett, M.D., and colleagues at Harvard University's School of Public Health in Boston, who found that *as little as one drink per day may raise a woman's risk of breast cancer by 60 percent.* Many questions remain about the association of alcohol and breast cancer risk. Compounding the issue is evidence suggesting that moderate amounts of alcohol (one or two drinks per day) may protect against heart disease, which causes ten times more deaths than breast cancer. Until we know more, most experts recommend that women who are at especially high risk for breast cancer—those who are obese, who have had few children, who were first pregnant when they were older than age thirty, or whose mothers had breast cancer—abstain from drinking altogether, or at least curtail their alcohol consumption.

Another way to protect yourself is to engage in some kind of regular physical activity. Studies by Harvard University researcher Rose Frisch, Ph.D., have found that female athletes have about half the incidence of breast cancer and other cancers of the reproductive organs as sedentary women.

There's some evidence that taking a progestogen

along with estrogen may help protect women against breast cancer. In a nine-year study investigating the association between estrogen use and breast cancer risk, R. Don Gambrell, M.D., and colleagues at the Medical College of Georgia in Augusta, found that among the 3,940 women in the study, those who had taken a progestogen along with estrogen had the lowest incidence of cancer. In a twenty-two-year study conducted by Dr. Nachtigall at New York University Medical Center, none of the eighty-four women who took estrogen and progestogen developed breast cancer, while six of the eighty-four study participants who didn't take hormones developed breast cancer.

Of course, the earlier a breast cancer is detected and treated, the greater are the chances of a cure. In fact, *80 to 90 percent of breast cancers are cured when caught early*, which is why close surveillance of all women on hormone additive therapy is essential.

The best protection you have against breast cancer is literally in your own hands: More than 80 percent of breast lumps are found by patients themselves through breast self-examination. Studies have shown that women who practice BSE are diagnosed at an earlier stage of the cancer's development than those who don't. This translates into improved survival rates: Breast cancer patients who practice BSE have a 15 percent increased survival rate over those who don't.

BSE is most effective when it is done right—and regularly. If you don't routinely practice breast self-examination, ask your doctor to show you how, or follow the guide on page 153. Most major health organizations recommend that you examine your breasts once a month, but we recommend that you perform BSE once a week. Weekly BSE not only gets you into the habit of performing this essential examination, but also makes you more proficient at it. So make a habit of practicing BSE "Always on Sundays."

You should also have your breasts examined annually by your physician or another trained health care professional and you should most definitely have a yearly mammogram (a low-dose X ray of the breasts). *Mammograms can detect a breast lump up to two years before it can be felt by hand.*

The current data on breast cancer risk are not conclusive enough to change the way we prescribe postmenopausal hormones. But studies do point to the need for additional research. Until we know more, it's safe for women who would benefit most from postmenopausal hormones to take them, provided they're closely monitored. Our policy is to monitor carefully women with a family history of breast cancer (whose risk is about double that of women with a family history of breast cancer who don't take estrogen). Having fibrocystic breast disease (benign breast lumps) is not a reason to forego estrogen additive therapy, but may be a reason to use an added progestogen—even if you have had a hysterectomy.

Lung Cancer

Lung cancer is the leading cause of cancer death among women today, and cigarette smoking is largely responsible. In fact, there is a direct correlation between the number of women who started smoking after World War II and—twenty years later—the rise in lung cancer deaths.

Postmenopausal estrogen has not been associated

with an increase in lung cancer among women. But one published study has noted an increase in lung cancer among men being treated with estrogen for heart disease. These preliminary results leads to the suspicion that cigarette smokers who also take estrogen may be at an increased risk of developing lung cancer. Although no researchers have formally investigated the issue, we do know that the lungs contain a rich supply of estrogen receptors. It's possible that estrogen may act as a "Trojan horse," carrying the carbon residues from cigarette smoke into the lung cells and in this way helping to promote lung cancer.

Other Types of Cancer

If you have had melanoma (the most serious type of skin cancer), you should not take estrogen therapy, since melanoma may be fueled by estrogen. However, other types of cancer, including cancer of the colon and cervix, and most types of ovarian cancer are not a contraindication to estrogen therapy.

Other Complications of Hormone Additive Therapy

Hormone additive therapy has been associated with a few other complications, as well.

Gallstones: One or two studies have shown a slight increase in the risk of developing gallstones among women who take estrogen. However, it's still not clear whether the estrogen actually *caused* the development of gallstones. At any rate, this complication is very rare. If you or your physician suspect you may have gallstones, you may want to undergo an ultrasound scan of your gallbladder before beginning hormone additive therapy.

Liver disease: If you have significant hepatitis or suffered residual liver damage as a result of a past bout with hepatitis, we recommend the use of a patch, pellets, or some other nonoral form of estrogen that bypasses the liver altogether.

Who Should *Not* Take Hormones?

The list of women who *should not* take hormones is actually quite short. If you have unexplained vaginal bleeding, breast or endometrial cancer, or have had a recent heart attack, you definitely should not take hormones. If you've had ovarian cancer, you should check with your physician about taking estrogen. Some types of ovarian cancer have estrogen receptors and the cancer's recurrence or spread might be stimulated by the estrogen in hormone additive therapy.

Some women will need to be monitored more closely while taking hormone additive therapy, including women with seizure disorders, hypertension, benign fibroid tumors of the uterus, high blood cholesterol, migraine headaches, previous superficial blood clots in the legs (thrombophlebitis), endometriosis, and gallbladder disease.

Overall, the risks associated with hormone additive therapy are small. As you have seen, taking an added progestogen along with estrogen can actually *protect against* endometrial cancer. And for most women, the benefits of taking estrogen far outweigh the slightly increased risk of breast cancer. Any increased breast cancer risk associated with estrogen use can be reduced by eating a sensible, low-fat diet, exercising regularly, restricting alcohol consumption to a moderate level, regularly examining your breasts with BSE, and having yearly mammograms.

❦

CHAPTER 8

Pills, Patches, or Pellets: Your Choices for Hormone Therapy

A wide array of hormonal preparations is available today—from pills to patches to pellets. You should be aware, however, that all are not equal in terms of their effectiveness or potential side effects. Nor do all women respond to the same medication in the same way. Cost and convenience factor into the equation, too, particularly when you must take postmenopausal hormones for many years.

To get the most benefit from hormone additive therapy with the fewest side effects, you should first acquaint yourself with the various types of hormonal preparations available to you.

What Forms of Estrogen Are Currently Available?

As you have already seen, estrogen is one of the most effective ways to ease the physical discomforts of menopause and to help prevent heart disease and osteoporosis. Unlike birth control pills, which contain synthetic estrogens, most estrogens prescribed for menopausal women are "natural" estrogens, which are much safer and are associated with far fewer side effects. ("Natural" estrogens is actually a bit of a misnomer, since the most widely used, *conjugated equine estrogens*, come from horses, not humans.)

Estrogens can be administered in several different ways, and the route of administration sometimes *does* make a difference:

Oral Estrogen

The most commonly prescribed form of estrogen is oral estrogen, which is fairly easy to swallow in terms of cost and convenience. There are several types of oral preparations: *Conjugated equine estrogens* (Premarin) are derived from the urine of pregnant mares, and contain many different types of estrogen, some unique to horses. *Micronized estradiol* (Estrace), *esterified estrogen* (Estratab), and *estropipate* (Ogen), are considered "natural" estrogens because their chemical makeup closely resembles the estrogens in the human body. *Ethinyl estradiol* (Estinyl) and *quinestrol* (Estrovis) are synthetic hormones whose chemical structure is markedly different from that of human estrogens.

One potential drawback to oral estrogen is that it passes through the liver before entering your bloodstream. The liver acts on the estrogen in several ways. To begin with, all estrogens (except *ethinyl estradiol*, found in oral contraceptives) are converted to *estrone*, which is less potent than *estradiol*. (Before the estrone enters your cells, your body converts it back into estradiol.) Second, some of the estrogen is bound by proteins produced by the liver, rendering it incapable of entering your cells. Third, some of the estrogen is metabolized, or broken down by the liver.

Because of these changes, sometimes only from 5 to 45 percent of the oral estrogen you take may be "free" and therefore biologically active.

On the other hand, some oral estrogens which have been used now for fifty years, have stood the test of time. Virtually all of the scientific studies showing a beneficial effect of estrogen on bone mass and protection from cardiovascular disease in the United States have involved oral estrogen. Indeed, the fact that oral estrogen passes through the liver is one reason why it helps raise levels of protective HDL cholesterol. Newer forms of estrogen, such as the patch, still need to prove their ability to prevent fractures and protect against heart disease. (There's no reason to believe that these forms of estrogen won't be just as effective as oral estrogen.)

Transdermal Skin Patch

This is a paper-thin, half-dollar-size transparent oval patch with adhesive on one side. When placed on your skin (usually your lower abdomen or back), the patch slowly releases a small amount of estradiol each day. The estradiol is absorbed through the skin and directly into the bloodstream, thus bypassing the intestines and liver. With the patch and other nonoral forms of estrogen (discussed below) there's less binding, less breakdown of estrogen by the liver, and—theoretically —easier access of the hormone to the cell. As a result, these types of estrogen can be more potent than oral estrogen, and lower doses should be used.

The patch must be changed twice weekly. Your physician will usually prescribe the lower strength (.05 mg) first, increasing the dosage (to .10 mg) if your symptoms don't subside after a few months. (The patch

TABLE 8-1. How Various Estrogen Preparations Affect Estrogen Levels in Your Body

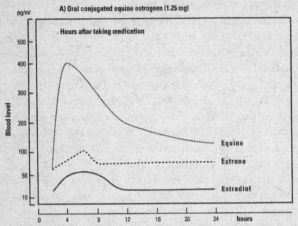

Chart adapted with permission from Whittaker, Paul G., "Metabolism of Oral Estrogen." *International Journal of Fertility*, 1986 (supplement), pages 21–28. Copyright © 1986 by U.S. International Foundation for Studies in Reproduction, Inc., Scandinavian Association for Studies in Fertility, and International Federation of Fertilities Societies.

can also be divided into quarters or halves for an even lower dose; however, your pharmacist will have to perform this task because a special cutter must be used to seal in the medication after the patch has been divided.)

One advantage of the estrogen patch is that the slow, steady release of estrogen into your bloodstream helps keep blood estrogen levels fairly stable, thus preventing the peaks and valleys in blood estrogen levels sometimes associated with pills (see Table 8-1). Another advantage is that you can't overdose.

The patch has a few disadvantages. Some 20 percent of women using the patch will experience a skin reaction. The estrogen in the patch may be poorly or inad-

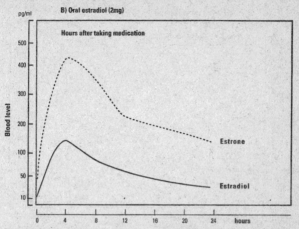

Chart adapted with permission from Kuhl, H. "Pharmacokinetics of Oestrogens and Progestogens." *Maturitas* 1990, Volume 12, pages 171–197. Copyright © 1990 by Elsevier Scientific Publishers Ireland Ltd.

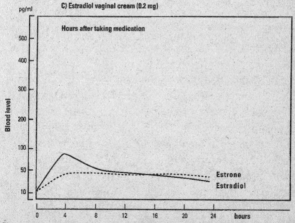

Chart adapted with permission from Rigg, Lee A., Hermann, Harold, and Yen, Samuel C. "Absorption of estrogens from vaginal creams. *The New England Journal of Medicine*, Vol. 298, No. 4, January 26, 1978, pages 195–197.

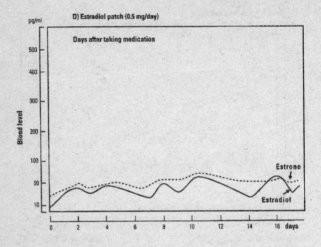

Chart adapted with permission from Powers, Marilou S., Schenkel, L., Darley, Paul E., Good, William R., Balestra, Joanne C., and Place, Virgil A. "Pharmacokinetics and Pharmacodynamics of transdermal dosage forms of 17beta-estradiol: Comparison with conventional oral estrogens used for hormone replacement." *American Journal of Obstetrics and Gynecology*, Vol. 152, No. 8, August 15, 1985, pages 1099–1106.

equately absorbed through the skin, especially in warm, humid climates. Also, the lower blood hormone levels associated with the patch may be inadequate protection against osteoporosis and heart disease for some women. (Your doctor can monitor your blood-estradiol levels to ensure that you are getting adequate protection against heart disease and osteoporosis.) Finally, some women may have trouble remembering to change the patch twice a week. It's best to establish a regular schedule (a calendar appears on the patch's packaging, making it easier to remember the schedule).

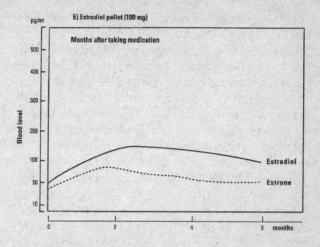

Chart adapted with permission from Thom, M. H., Collins, W. P. and Studol, J. W. W. "Hormonal Profiles in Postmenopausal Women after Therapy with Subcutaneous Implants." *British Journal of Obstetrics and Gynaecology.* April 1981, Vol. 88, pages 426–433.

Tips for Using the Skin Patch

•To help prevent skin irritation, rotate the areas to which you apply the patch. The best place to use the patch is on the back just above the buttock.

•If skin irritation occurs, move the patch to another site. Your doctor may prescribe a low-dose steroid cream to clear up persistent skin irritations.

•If the patch falls off in the shower or while exercising, leave it off until after you've finished, dry the skin thoroughly, then reapply the patch.

Vaginal Creams (Estrace, Estraguard, Ogen, Ortho Dienestrol, Premarin)

Estrogen cream is ideal for women whose main complaint is vaginal dryness or urinary symptoms because the cream goes right to the heart of the problem—the estrogen-deprived vaginal and urethral tissues. Because the cream is applied directly to the tissues that need it most, many women think of vaginal estrogen as a "local" treatment that is "safer" than other forms of estrogen that circulate throughout the body. After all, estrogen cream affects only the vaginal and urethral tissues and doesn't circulate in the bloodstream, right? Not exactly. What most women don't realize is that estrogen cream is quickly absorbed through the vaginal walls into the bloodstream, so, in effect, this "local" treatment can (if large enough quantities are used) have a systemic effect. This isn't a problem for most women. In fact, the vagina's ability to absorb estrogen can actually be a therapeutic advantage for some women (see vaginal use of oral tablets, below). But women who wish to minimize their exposure to systemic estrogen, such as those with a family history of breast cancer, could be getting a bigger dose of estrogen than they bargained for when using estrogen creams.

When used in reduced dosages (for instance ¼-applicatorful two to three times per week), estrogen creams are perfectly safe, and the amount of estrogen absorbed from the vagina into the bloodstream is quite low (see Table 8-1). You can further reduce the amount of estrogen absorbed by massaging a small amount of cream into the vagina with your finger. Even if you have a family history of breast cancer, you can still use vaginal creams. (We recommend that women with a family history of breast cancer use Estrace cream, since it contains only the hormone estradiol and your blood hormone levels can be easily monitored while you're using the cream.)

A plastic applicator is used to insert the cream into the vagina. Applying the cream just before bedtime increases absorption. As with most hormone preparations, how much cream you'll need to take depends on your reasons for using it (see chapter 9, "A Symptoms Guide to Hormone Additive Therapy").

The biggest drawback to creams is that some women find them messy. Newer forms of vaginal estrogen, many of which may be available in the U.S. within the next five years (see page 113), should help solve this problem. Until some of these newer preparations become available, wear a sanitary napkin or panty liner to protect your clothes while using vaginal creams.

Vaginal Use of Oral Tablets

An alternative to oral estrogen for women who can't use the skin patch involves placing half a tablet of oral estradiol (Estrace) into the vagina every two to three days. This treatment results in moderate blood levels of estrogen that may last for up to thirty-six hours. Since only 25 to 50 percent of the usual oral dosage is used, this method is more cost-effective than oral estrogen.

The only disadvantages are that you must break the tablets in half yourself and, because the tablets are colored purple, they may stain your undergarments. (Wearing a panty shield or panty liner helps solve this problem.)

Estradiol Pellets

Estrogen-containing pellets—each about the size of a saccharine tablet—can be injected in the fat tissue just under the skin (usually in the lower abdomen or buttock) by a physician. Once injected, the pellet slowly releases its medication into the bloodstream and is absorbed by the body.

The chief advantage of this method is that one or two pellets containing 25 milligrams of estradiol each provides steady blood levels of estrogen for three to four months after you receive it. The pellets are usually prescribed for women who have experienced little or no relief of their symptoms from oral estrogen or those who experienced side effects from oral estrogen. (Testosterone pellets may be used along with the estrogen for women who experience a decreased sex drive or other problems that respond well to androgen therapy; for more on androgens, see page 119.)

The main drawback to the pellet is that it is difficult to remove if you experience any unwanted side effects. (This is rare, since most women using the pellets experience *relief* from their symptoms after finding oral estrogen ineffective.) Since it is also difficult to tell when the pellet has been spent, your blood hormone levels will have to be monitored more closely while using this form of estrogen therapy. And, of course, you will have to see your physician and undergo a minor surgical procedure each time your supply of estrogen runs out.

Intramuscular Injection

Several injectable forms of estrogen, lasting up to four weeks, are available. However, injections are associated with peaks and valleys in blood estrogen levels, and for this reason are not usually recommended. If you do receive injections, your blood hormone levels will have to be frequently monitored, and the dose of estrogen adjusted accordingly.

What Forms of Estrogen Will Be Available in the Near Future?

Several new forms of estrogen are now being investigated in the United States, and may be available within the next five years.

Vaginal Tablet
An estrogen tablet with the unique ability to coat the vaginal walls is now used in Europe, and is currently under investigation in the United States. The estrogen in the tablet is not absorbed through the vaginal walls or into the bloodstream, so the therapeutic effects of the drug remain localized in the vagina. For this reason, it may be safer for some women than vaginal creams, most of which *do* raise blood estrogen levels, depending on the dosage.

Estradiol Ring
This thin, flexible rubber ring is worn much like a diaphragm in the vagina, where it gradually releases a small amount of estrogen. The ring can be left in place during intercourse and can be easily removed to regulate or change the drug dosage being given. (Some researchers are also experimenting with a vaginal ring containing a combination of estrogen and progesterone to help protect the endometrial lining from overstimulation by estrogen alone.) The main advantage is that the ring is not as messy as vaginal creams.

Gel
A new estradiol-containing gel now available in Europe may make estrogen additive therapy as simple as using a moisturizing cream or lotion every day. The gel,

which is squeezed out of a tube in measured doses, may be applied to the arms, shoulders, waist, thighs, or other parts of the body (except for the breasts) in much the same way as you'd apply a moisturizing cream or lotion. The gel dries rapidly (usually within two minutes), leaves no sticky residue, and has no odor.

The gel provides the same steady blood hormone levels as the patch, but the overall blood levels of estradiol are higher among gel users than patch users.

What Forms of Progestogen Are Currently Available?

Progestogens are prescribed to prevent overstimulation of the uterine lining by estrogen and hence help protect against the development of endometrial cancer among women who still have an intact uterus. *Women who have had a hysterectomy don't need to take a progestogen, even if their ovaries remain intact (see "Who Needs Progestogen.")*

Oral Progestogens
Most progestogens today are given orally in one of three dosing regimens:

1. If you take estrogen for twenty-five days, you'll take an added progestogen for days fifteen through twenty-five, followed by five days of no medication, which is what's known as a *twenty-five-day cyclic regimen.*

2. If you take an estrogen every day without a break, you'll take an added progestogen during the first two weeks of every month, which is known as a *continuous cyclic regimen.*

3. You may also take an estrogen and a progestogen every day, in a *continuous combined regimen*.

All regimens protect equally well against endometrial cancer. However, there are several chemically different types of oral progestogens, and sometimes the choice of progestogen you use does make a difference.

Who Needs Progestogen?

If you have an intact uterus	Yes
If you have had a hysterectomy (uterus removed but ovaries intact)	No
If you have had a hysterectomy and oophorectomy (uterus and ovaries removed)	No
If you have had an oophorectomy (one or both ovaries removed, uterus intact)	Yes

---

Medroxyprogesterone acetate (Provera, Curretab, Amen): This is the most widely used progestogen in the United States, and has one of the longest track records for safety and effectiveness. For this reason, your physician may recommend that you begin hormone additive therapy with this type of progestogen. This is particularly true if you have a past history of breast problems (such as fibrocystic breast disease). Some physicians believe this type of progestogen may inhibit benign breast disease and possibly protect against breast cancer. However, these progestogens may not be the best choice for women being treated for mood swings and other estrogen-dependent psychological symptoms, since studies have linked Provera with an increase in moodiness and depression.

19 Nortestosterone derivatives (Aygestin, Norlutate, Norlutin, Ovrette): These progestogens are fairly potent, but if used in low enough doses, they don't affect blood lipids and, because they are more potent, may better protect the endometrium than other progestogens.

Your physician may recommend these progestogens if you have a past history of heavy or prolonged menstrual periods (they help reduce bleeding somewhat), or if you are taking estrogen to help relieve menopause-related emotional symptoms.

Megesterol acetate (Megace): This progestogen is used primarily for the treatment of breast and endometrial cancers. However, Megace is also a good treatment for hot flashes among women with breast and endometrial cancer. The drug should be used in collaboration with an oncologist (cancer specialist) to ensure you get the proper dosage of the medication. If the cancer is estrogen- or progesterone-sensitive, you'll need to take a full chemotherapeutic dose.

Micronized oral progesterone: This formulation of natural progesterone doesn't adversely affect blood lipids and doesn't cause the mood swings associated with some synthetic hormones. While the drug has not yet received approval from the U.S. Food and Drug Administration, your physician may be able to obtain it from independent pharmacists.

Progestasert IUD

The progestogen-containing intrauterine device, Progestasert, may be an ideal way for postmenopausal women taking estrogen to protect themselves against endometrial cancer. The IUD, inserted into the uterus by a physician, slowly releases a small amount of progestogen. Since the progesterone is administered locally, it doesn't adversely affect blood lipids.

What Forms of Progestogen Will Be Available in the Near Future?

Most of the progestogens used today can produce side effects similar to those associated with the male hormone androgen, including acne, weight gain, and negative changes in blood cholesterol levels. However, three new types of progestogens being investigated in the United States and Europe, *gestodene*, *desogestrel*, and *norgestimate* have few androgenlike properties, so these side effects are unlikely to occur. A transdermal skin patch containing both estrogen and a progesterone may also reduce the negative side effects of progestogen on blood lipids.

If I Take Progestogen Along with Estrogen, Will I Get Monthly Periods Again?

This is one of the more pressing questions of women who must take a combination of estrogen and progestogen to protect against endometrial cancer, particularly when the cessation of monthly bleeding is seen as one of the *benefits* of menopause. Indeed, resumption of menstruallike bleeding is the chief reason women give for *not* taking hormones prescribed to them, or for stopping hormone additive therapy soon after they've begun taking it.

Actually, the bleeding you experience is *not* a real menstrual period in the true sense of the word, since it is the shedding of an artificially stimulated endometrium. *How much* bleeding you expect and *when* you can expect it depends on which one of the three estrogen-progestogen regimens you take.

1. *Twenty-five-day cyclic regimen.* If you take estrogen for twenty-five days, an added progestogen for days fifteen through twenty-five, followed by five days of no medication, you can expect to experience some bleeding during the five day interval in which you take no hormones.

2. *Continuous cyclic regimen.* If you take an estrogen every day without a break, along with an added progestogen during the first two weeks of every month, you will experience some bleeding during the middle of the month.

3. *Continuous combined regimen.* If you take an estrogen and a progestogen every day, you may experience some irregular bleeding and light spotting for the first four months. (Sixty percent of women on this regimen won't bleed at all during the first four to six months.) After six months, few women will experience any bleeding.

For most women, the menstrual effects of combined estrogen-progestogen therapy are minimal. (A minority of women may experience heavy bleeding, menstrual cramps, and pain; See chapter 10 for ways to alleviate these symptoms.) Keep in mind, too, that the benefits of taking hormone additive therapy—prevention of fractures ten years from now, for instance, or protection from cardiovascular disease—far outweigh the minor inconvenience of menstruallike bleeding.

What Forms of Androgen Are Currently Available?

Your body continues to produce low levels of the "male" hormone testosterone as well as other androgens, even after menopause. Low androgen levels have been associated with such menopause-related symptoms as depression, headaches, sex drive, and even bone loss.

Prescription androgens are occasionally used to help alleviate some of these symptoms. If you continue to have symptoms on estrogen therapy alone, your practitioner may recommend that you take an androgen along with your estrogen. Preliminary evidence suggests that androgens may help in the following ways:

•**An increased sense of well-being.** Several studies have found that women who take androgens along with estrogens get more than relief from such menopausal symptoms as hot flashes. In a study by Barbara Sherwin, Ph.D., at McGill University in Montreal, those who took an androgen-estrogen combination reported a greater sense of well-being and energy than those who took estrogen alone. Another study investigating the mood-enhancing effects of testosterone found that those who received estrogen and androgens felt more composed, elated, and energetic than those who were given estrogen alone. Our own 1982 study of the effects of aging and menopause on women buoys these findings. In our study, higher levels of testosterone in postmenopausal women who were not taking hormones were associated with an increased feeling of well-being.

•**Improved sex drive.** While estrogen can help relieve painful intercourse as a result of menopause-related changes in the vagina, several studies now show that testosterone is critical for maintaining desire and interest in sex. Women who take androgens have higher levels of sexual desire, sexual arousal, and fantasy than women who receive estrogen alone or a placebo. Androgen-users also make love more often and have more orgasms than nonusers.

•**Fewer headaches.** Women who suffer from hormonal headaches (usually migraine headaches triggered by estrogen therapy; see page 140) often find relief by taking androgens along with estrogen.

•**Relief from depression.** Androgen-estrogen combinations work even better than estrogen alone in alleviating depression associated with the hormonal changes of menopause. (Androgens *do not* boost the mood of women suffering from true clinical depression, however.)

•**Increased bone mass.** Adding androgens to estrogen therapy may help prevent bone loss, possibly by enhancing the effects of estrogen. Women with vertebral crush fractures reportedly have lower testosterone levels than women without fractures. Columbia University's Robert Lindsay, M.D., showed that the more rapid bone loss in the early menopausal years is associated with low blood levels of estrogen *and* the androgen *androstenedione*. Others have found virtually no bone loss—and no new collapsed vertebrae in osteoporosis patients who received estrogen and testosterone for thirty years. In a recent study of ours, women taking estrogen alone maintained bone mass in the lumbar spine, while those who took an estrogen along with testosterone experienced a 3 percent *increase* in bone mass after twelve months, and a 4 percent increase after twenty-four months.

While some researchers worried that giving androgens to women would raise their blood cholesterol levels (and heart disease risk), to date, most studies involving estrogen combined with a nonoral androgen have found little or no change in blood lipids. However, oral androgens may reduce protective high density lipoproteins.

On the other hand, oral androgens appear to reduce triglycerides, and may help offset the *rise* in blood triglycerides that is often triggered by oral estrogen. In a recent study we conducted, women taking an estrogen-androgen combination experienced a 20 percent decrease in blood triglycerides. So there may actually be a role for androgens in the prevention of cardiovascular disease.

Androgens aren't without side effects, however. Your skin may become more oily, increasing the possibility of developing acne. Mild hirsutism, or hair growth (including facial hair), occurs in about 15 to 20 percent of patients. Sometimes, simply taking a lower dosage of androgens helps alleviate these symptoms. Taking the diuretic *spironolactone* (Aldactone, Aldactazine) often helps, too.

You should be aware that androgens *don't* protect against overstimulation of the uterine lining by estrogen. So if you have an intact uterus and are being treated with an estrogen-androgen combination, you should also take a progestogen to guard against endometrial cancer.

Androgens are available in the form of oral tablets, injections, and pellets.

Oral Androgens
Tablets containing 1.25 milligrams to 2.5 milligrams of methyltestosterone are taken daily, and are usually taken along with an oral estrogen from the first through the twenty-fifth day of the month (to minimize side effects).

Androgen Injection
A long-acting form of testosterone may be given by injection. The dose is usually 50 to 75 milligrams of testosterone every four weeks. Because blood levels of testosterone are high right after you receive the injection, then decline over the four-week interval, you may experience a gradual decline in its therapeutic effects over time.

Implants
Testosterone pellets may be used along with estrogen pellets (two estrogen pellets with one testosterone pellet). Effects usually last from three to six months.

Ointment
Testosterone propionate ointment can be applied locally to the clitoris.

What Estrogen/Androgen Combinations Are Currently Available?

Oral
Several estrogen-androgen tablets are available in this country. Some (Estratest and Estratest H.S.) contain es-

terified estrogens and methyltestosterone. Combination products of conjugated estrogens are also available (Premarin with Methyltestosterone), but they are not as well-balanced as those containing esterified estrogens.

Injection
A combination estrogen-androgen injectable, Depo-Testadiol, usually relieves symptoms for four weeks.

What About Generic Estrogen Preparations?

Generic drugs are usually less expensive than their name-brand counterparts, and there are generic equivalents to many of the commonly prescribed estrogen preparations, particularly conjugated estrogens. You should be aware, however, that most generic conjugated estrogens contain fewer estrogens than name brands. And while generic preparations initially are absorbed more rapidly into the bloodstream (resulting in higher peak blood levels of estrogen), after about eight hours the levels of estrogen circulating in the bloodstream for generic brands tend to be lower than those for name brands. It's still not known whether these differences affect the overall efficacy of generic drugs. Until we know more, we recommend that you request name-brand drugs from your pharmacist instead of generic brands.

Now that you know what's available to you, let's take a look at which hormonal preparation—or combination of preparations—works best for your particular needs.

CHAPTER 9

❧

A Symptoms Guide to Hormone Additive Therapy

The type and amount of estrogen and progestogen you take depends largely on your reason for taking it. Here are some general guidelines to help you and your doctor decide which hormonal preparation will work best for you.

Which Hormone Therapies Are Best for Which Menopausal Symptoms?

If You Have Hot Flashes and Sleep Disruptions
Most types of estrogen (pill, patch, pellet, or injection) work equally well in relieving hot flashes. (Estrogen creams generally are not prescribed for these symptoms.) Your physician will prescribe the lowest possible dose of estrogen to control your symptoms.

Since peak blood estrogen levels occur from four to six hours after taking oral estrogen, you should take your medication just before bedtime. If you take your estrogen in the morning, you may continue to be bothered by early morning awakenings and night sweats because by this time, blood estrogen levels have fallen.

Some women may have to take oral estrogen twice a day: once in the morning and once at night.

It may take three to four weeks before you feel the full effects of estrogen on your symptoms. If after three months your symptoms still haven't subsided, your physician will gradually increase the dosage as needed, or change to another route of administration.

If your uterus is intact, you'll have to take a progestogen, either cyclically or continuously, along with the estrogen.

Three to five years is the average length of time that hormones are used to control hot flashes. However, in some women, symptoms persist—and treatment may be required—for many years. Some 30 percent of women over age sixty need hormone additive therapy for hot flashes. Therapy generally is tapered off over a few months, then stopped altogether.

You should note that the low dose of estrogen used to relieve hot flashes may be too low for protection against cardiovascular disease or osteoporosis. If one of your objectives is to protect your heart or bones, you may need to take a larger dose for a longer period of time. Check with your physician.

If You Have Psychological Symptoms

Systemic estrogens (pills, pellets, or patches) work best. Some women may find that nonoral types of estrogen (pellets or patches) work better than pills, since there's less of a binding effect on the drug by the liver, which increases the bioavailability and effectiveness of the drug. If you are sensitive to fluctuations in hormone levels, the patch and pellets also provide more stable blood estrogen levels.

Progestogens are another matter: If you need to take

a progestogen, some—particularly *medroxyprogesterone acetate* (Amen, Curretab, Provera)—may aggravate or induce depression and other PMS-like psychological symptoms. If this is the case, you could ask your physician to prescribe *19-nortestosterone derivatives* in appropriate reduced dosages (Aygestin, Norlutate, Norlutin, Ovrette, Micronor), which are less likely to trigger depression. Oral micronized progesterone may in fact be the best.

If You Have Headaches

Continuous estrogen therapy with oral estrogen may help relieve migraine headaches. If oral estrogen doesn't improve your migraines, often the estrogen patch or estrogen pellets will, since these forms of estrogen are associated with more steady blood estrogen levels. On the other hand, cyclic therapy, in which you take estrogen for three weeks, then stop taking the medication for a week, results in a period of "estrogen withdrawal" that has been associated with an increase in migraine headaches. You and your physician may have to experiment with various forms of estrogen before finding one that works for you.

Adding an androgen to postmenopausal estrogen therapy may help, too. In one study by R. Don Gambrell, Jr., M.D., a gynecologist at the Medical College of Georgia in Augusta, 20 percent of patients who had headaches reported improvement after treatment with estrogen pellets alone. However, 60 percent reported improvement with the combination of estrogen plus testosterone.

Progestogens, which are usually given along with estrogen to protect against overstimulation of the uterine lining, may aggravate migraines. Some women whose headaches are relieved with continuous estrogen therapy alone find that the migraines and mood swings return when they take a progestogen cyclically along with estrogen. If progestogens are a problem, your physician may first recommend that you change the type of progestogen you are taking. If this doesn't work, he or she may reduce the dosage of progestogen to the lowest possible amount needed to protect the uterine lining. If headaches persist, switching to oral micronized progesterone or a progesterone IUD may solve the problem.

If You Have Vaginal Dryness

Vaginal creams are the treatment of choice for vaginal dryness and urethral and bladder-related symptoms. Systemic estrogens (oral, patch, pellets) are not as effective in relieving vaginal symptoms. In one study we conducted in conjunction with Gloria Bachmann, M.D., at the University of Medicine and Dentistry of New Jersey in New Brunswick, 44 percent of women taking oral estrogen still complained of vaginal dryness.

A low dose (one-fourth to one-half an applicatorful) is usually prescribed because estrogen is well-absorbed from the vagina. (Using your finger to massage a small amount of estrogen into the vagina helps reduce absorption of the cream into the bloodstream.) You should use estrogen creams two to three times a week for three to six months. You may need a "maintenance" dose of estrogen cream twice a week thereafter.

If You Have Urethral Syndrome

Vaginal estrogen creams are often recommended for women with urethral syndrome, inflammation of the urethra that causes such symptoms as increased frequency of urination and a sense of urgency. The dosage is one-quarter to one-half an applicatorful (placed in the vagina) three times a week for three to six months. Massaging a small amount of cream into the vaginal walls with your finger every night also helps.

Which Hormone Therapies Are Best for Preventing Which Types of Cardiovascular Disease?

Hormone therapy for the prevention of cardiovascular disease should be tailored to women who are, for one reason or other, at increased risk of developing heart and vascular problems.

If You Have High Blood Pressure
As mentioned in chapter 5, oral estrogen actually *lowers* blood pressure. For the minority of women whose blood pressure rises after beginning hormone therapy, or for women whose hypertension is related to the hormone *renin*, the estrogen patch should be used.

If You Have Diabetes
If your blood triglycerides are elevated, you should use the patch, since oral estrogen may increase blood triglycerides. If your levels of HDL cholesterol are not too low, you could consider using an oral estrogen-androgen combination, since the androgens appear to offset the rise in blood triglycerides associated with oral estrogens. Otherwise, oral estrogen is fine because it actually *lowers* blood sugar levels.

If You Have a History of Blood Clots

Women with previous deep venous thrombosis *can* take estrogen, particularly if the blood clot was from a non-recurring cause. (For instance, a woman who developed phlebitis after a caesarean section twenty years ago might safely use hormone additive therapy.)

What kind of estrogen is best? If you had a remote deep venous thrombosis, the type of estrogen you use makes no difference. If you have recently developed a blood clot from a nonrecurring cause (for instance, after a hysterectomy), your first choice should probably be the skin patch, which has less of an effect on coagulation factors produced by the liver.

Should you stop estrogen additive therapy before surgery? It's probably not necessary, but it may be prudent to do so for one month prior to surgery. Immediately after surgery, you should use the skin patch.

A precautionary note: All women with a history of blood clots should be closely monitored. Your physician can test for levels of fibrinogen, the activity of anticoagulants, such as antithrombin III, and the overall marker of your blood's ability to clot—prothrombin time. If you have a history of blood clots we recommend that you take a junior aspirin (60 milligrams) every three days. Aspirin helps decrease platelet adhesiveness and encourages dilation of the blood vessels. (You should take aspirin regularly only while under a doctor's supervision. See page 72.) You should also exercise, which increases blood flow through your body and may raise levels of certain anticoagulants. Moreover, *you should not smoke*. Cigarette smoking increases the "stickiness" of blood platelets, decreasing clotting time, increasing blood thickness, and increasing the likelihood that a blood clot will form. Plus, cigarette smoking appears to damage the lining of arteries and depresses the production of the anticoagulant prostacyclin by the blood vessel wall, both of which may increase the risk that a blood clot will form.

If You Have High Blood Cholesterol and/or a Family History of Cardiovascular Disease

Most of the studies showing a protective effect are based on the use of oral conjugated estrogens (Premarin). We found that *estropipate* (Ogen) was also highly effective in reducing blood cholesterol, especially among women with elevated cholesterol (above 260 mg/dl). After twelve months, total cholesterol of the women taking Ogen in our study fell 3.4 percent, LDL cholesterol dropped 8.3 percent, and HDL cholesterol rose 9.7 percent. If you have high cholesterol and decreased HDL cholesterol, you should consider taking oral Premarin, Ogen, Estrace, Estratab or other equivalents.

If your triglycerides are elevated, however, the patch may be a better choice, as oral estrogens may raise triglycerides. (If you have elevated triglycerides *and* fairly high levels of HDL-cholesterol, your physician may recommend an estrogen-androgen combination. Oral androgens have been found to lower triglycerides.)

As for progestogens, very low doses of *19-nortestosterone* or *oral micronized progesterone* are preferable because they have been shown to have the least effect on blood lipids. You should take the minimum dose needed to protect against endometrial cancer. You should also consider a *cyclic* rather than a *continuous* regimen of progestogen, since this further limits the amount of time you are exposed to progestogen.

(Note: The transdermal estrogen patch also alters blood lipids, but usually only after four to six months of treatment. The main positive effect of the patch is to lower LDL cholesterol levels, rather than increase protective HDL cholesterol levels. So if your HDL levels are low, in our opinion you must use oral estrogen.)

If You Have Established Coronary Heart Disease
It is not known if hormone therapy will be useful for women with established coronary heart disease. Hormone additive therapy may be a useful adjunct to other treatments, such as angioplasty. And since estrogen raises HDL cholesterol and lowers LDL cholesterol, it can be used in the treatment of high blood cholesterol (*hypercholesterolemia*). Of course, if you have high cholesterol levels, you should also eat a low-fat diet and exercise regularly. You may also need to take specific cholesterol-lowering drugs.

Which Hormone Therapies Are Best for Preventing Osteoporosis?

As a rule, if you have relatively normal bone mass (that is, any bone loss of less than 10 to 15 percent of the average bone mass of younger women), you can choose the type of estrogen and its route of administration. If you have low bone mass (a loss of more than 30 percent that of young women), we recommend oral estrogen, especially conjugated equine estrogens, since their ability to maintain bone mass has been better documented than that of the patch or other forms of estrogen.

The type of oral estrogen used doesn't make much difference so long as the dose is adequate. Here are the minimum doses for the most widely prescribed oral estrogen preparations:

Premarin	0.625 to 0.9 mg/day
Estrace	1 to 2 mg/day
Ogen	1.25 mg/day
Estratab	0.625 mg to 1.25 mg/day
Estinyl	20 micrograms/day

How long will you need to take hormones? It depends on how much bone mass you have to start with. If you are taking hormones to maintain relatively normal bone mass, you may take hormone therapy for ten to fifteen years, up to age sixty-five. If you have established osteoporosis or are at very high risk of developing osteoporosis, we recommend that you take hormones for the rest of your life, provided you have no contraindications, you don't experience any serious side effects during your treatment, and you undergo regular tests for breast and endometrial cancer. Why so long? When you stop taking hormone therapy, you could experience a substantial decrease in bone density.

Again, if you have experienced a natural menopause and your uterus is intact, you should take a progestogen along with estrogen to protect against endometrial cancer. An added progestogen may also help to add bone mass.

When deciding which method of hormone additive therapy is best for you, you will of course want to choose the most effective method for your particular needs. But you should also consider which method would be most convenient for you. Too often, women stop taking hormone therapy because the method they're using becomes burdensome in one way or another. If one form of hormone therapy becomes problematic for you, try another. Together, you and your physician should be able to find a perfect fit.

CHAPTER 10

❋

Hormones: How Will You Know If They're Working ... And Whether They're Safe for You?

If you decide to take hormone therapy, you should be monitored regularly by your physician for three reasons: to determine the effectiveness of the treatment, to ensure your safety, and to alleviate any side effects you may experience.

How to Judge the Effectiveness of Your Hormone Therapy

Remember: Estrogen works only for as long as you take it. When you stop taking estrogen, bone loss may resume, cholesterol levels may rise, and some women may experience hot flashes and other menopausal symptoms once again. (Hot flashes usually abate if hormone additive therapy is gradually tapered off.)

How will you know whether hormone therapy is working? It depends on your reason for using it.

If You Take Hormones to Treat Menopausal Symptoms

You will know whether hormone therapy is working to relieve hot flashes and other symptoms of menopause simply by the way you feel. If your symptoms persist, you may need a larger dose of estrogen. Or you may want to try a different route of administration.

Your physician can use more objective tests, such as vaginal pH and the maturation index of cells in the vaginal walls, to monitor the effectiveness of estrogen creams in the treatment of atrophic vaginitis.

If You Take Hormones to Prevent Heart Disease

Levels of total cholesterol, HDL cholesterol, LDL cholesterol, triglycerides, and the ratio of HDL to total cholesterol can be used as a gauge of whether hormone therapy is conferring protection against heart disease. We recommend that you undergo a lipid profile every other year after starting hormone additive therapy if your blood cholesterol levels are normal, and once a year if you have high cholesterol (above 240 mg/dl) high LDL cholesterol (above 140 mg/dl) or low HDL cholesterol (below 40 mg/dl).

If You Take Hormones to Prevent Osteoporosis

Having your bone density tested using dual energy X-ray absorptiometry (DEXA), a method capable of measuring the bone density of the wrist, hip and spine, is an ideal way to monitor how well hormone therapy is working. A simple urine test that monitors the ratio of calcium to creatinine (a by-product of metabolism) can also be used to monitor the effectiveness of your treatment. A blood test that measures levels of alkaline phosphatase and can tell whether new bone formation has been stimulated may also be helpful. Other tests now being developed may soon be available, as well. Ask your doctor.

Are the Hormones You Take Actually Being Used by Your Body?

Every woman responds a little differently to hormone therapy. If you don't respond to treatment, a blood test can detect the levels of estrogen (estradiol and estrone) circulating in your bloodstream and determine whether your body is absorbing the drugs you are taking. Blood estrogen levels don't always tell the whole story, however. Sometimes, estrogen circulating in the bloodstream can be "bound" by proteins and is not biologically available. Therefore, in addition to blood hormone tests, your physician may also measure levels of FSH (follicle stimulating hormone) to determine the biological efficacy of the hormones you're taking. High levels of FSH indicate that while estrogen may be absorbed into the bloodstream, most of the estrogen is not available in a form your body can use; what we call the "estrogen binding syndrome." Often, switching the route of administration (from pills to patch, or to vaginal use of pills, for instance) will help improve the biological activity of the drug.

How Do I Know My Hormone Therapy Is Safe?

As we mentioned earlier, the addition of a progestogen to estrogen therapy provides ample protection against endometrial cancer. Nevertheless, it's a good idea for you to be monitored for possible signs of endometrial and—until we know more about the effects of post-menopausal estrogens on your risk—breast cancer. We recommend that you periodically undergo the following tests:

Endometrial Sampling

This test involves removing a small sample of endometrial tissue from the uterus and examining it under a microscope to check for any abnormalities, such as *hyperplasia* (overgrowth of cells, or precancerous cells). The test is often recommended annually for women taking hormone additive therapy to ensure that the endometrial lining isn't being overstimulated by estrogen, and *any* time a woman taking hormone additive therapy experiences an abnormal bleeding pattern.

During the test, your physician will insert a long, narrow plastic or metal suctioning device, or *cannula*, through the cervix and into the uterus. The device is then used to suction out a small sample of the endometrial lining. The test itself usually causes mild cramping and discomfort, which can often be relieved by taking a nonsteroidal anti-inflammatory agent, such as aspirin or ibuprofen (Advil, Nuprin, Motrin IB) *an hour before* the procedure. You may also experience light vaginal bleeding for a day or two following the sampling procedure.

Your physician may use any one of a number of cannulas to take a sample of the endometrium; most differ only in the manner in which suction is produced. However, one of the newer devices, the Pipelle, is associated with less cramping and discomfort, mostly because it is much smaller in diameter than some of the other devices.

Some physicians recommend a baseline evaluation of

the endometrium before starting hormone additive therapy. Others (ourselves included) prefer to wait until after you've taken hormones for three months. This allows you time to adjust to the medication and gives your physician a chance to determine what effect the drug regimen has on your endometrium.

Ultrasound

If your cervical canal is tightly narrowed (*stenosed*), or if you are extremely sensitive to pain, your physician may instead use ultrasound to measure the thickness of your uterine lining. This is a painless procedure that takes about ten minutes. The test may be performed either abdominally or vaginally. During an abdominal examination, you lie on your back on an examining table and an oil or gel is spread over your abdomen. The practitioner moves a hand-held ultrasound probe slowly across your abdomen. The probe emits sound waves to project an image of your uterus on a video screen.

Since the abdominal ultrasound requires that you have a full bladder, which can be somewhat uncomfortable, many women prefer the vaginal ultrasound examination. During this examination, a narrow ultrasound probe is gently placed into the vagina.

An endometrial thickness of less than 5 millimeters is considered normal. If your uterine lining is more than 5 millimeters thick, additional tests, such as hysteroscopy or dilatation and curettage (D&C), may be required.

One of the drawbacks to ultrasound is that it doesn't provide an actual tissue sample that can be inspected under a microscope. However, a new color Doppler ultrasound may be even more accurate than the current method of measuring uterine thickness.

Regular Breast Examinations

We recommend weekly breast self-examinations (for instance, "Always on Sundays") to get you into the habit of performing these lifesaving examinations (see page 153 for directions on how to perform BSE), and also to give you more experience in performing the test, which ultimately makes the test more accurate. You may also want to consider having a breast examination by a health care professional every six months. And you should *definitely* undergo yearly mammograms.

Managing the Minor Side Effects of Hormone Therapy

Most minor side effects of hormone therapy are rare. When they do occur, bothersome side effects can often be ameliorated by changing the form of estrogen or progestogen you use or altering the dosing schedule (how much you take and when).

Discomforts Associated with Menstruallike Bleeding

For most women taking combined estrogen-progestogen therapy, menstrual bleeding is minimal. A minority of women, however, may experience heavy bleeding, menstrual cramps, and pain. These discomforts can usually be relieved by taking an anti-inflammatory, prostaglandin-inhibiting pain reliever, such as *ibuprofen* (Advil, Nuprin, Medipren, or the prescription brand Motrin), *naproxen* (Anaprox), or *mefenamic acid* (Ponstel). In addition to relieving pain, these drugs may decrease heavy bleeding by 50 percent.

If you do experience fairly heavy bleeding and use

tampons, be aware that some superabsorbency tampons have been associated with an increased risk of a potentially life-threatening bacterial infection known as toxic shock syndrome (TSS)—the greater the absorbency, the greater the risk. To reduce your risk, use the least absorbent tampon for your needs (the tampon's absorbency is now listed on the package) and change your tampon regularly (at least every four hours). You should see your physician immediately if, while using tampons, you suddenly develop a high fever, vomiting, diarrhea, or muscle pain, especially if these symptoms are accompanied by a sunburnlike rash.

Weight Gain

Some women may gain weight after beginning hormone therapy, but our research and that of others has shown that the average weight gain is only about five pounds—*if you gain any weight at all*. If you do gain weight after beginning hormone therapy, try readjusting your metabolic balance by eating less food and exercising more. If the weight you gain is mostly fluid, your physician may recommend that you take a diuretic.

Gastrointestinal Problems

Nausea and stomach upset may occur with some types of oral estrogens. These symptoms can be relieved by taking your pill with a little bit of food. (Note: Taking hormones with food enhances their absorption into the bloodstream.) If that doesn't help, you can change the type of oral estrogen you take, or switch to one of the nonoral types.

Breast Tenderness

If you notice increased breast tenderness after beginning hormone additive therapy, you may find relief by changing the way in which you take the hormone (switching to a Monday-through-Friday regimen, rather than taking the drug seven days a week, for instance). Decreasing the dosage to the bare minimum required to treat your condition may help, too. Your physician may recommend that you try a diuretic, an estrogen-androgen combination, or Tamoxifen (a drug used in the treatment of breast cancer), which sometimes helps to reduce breast tenderness. Cutting back on caffeine often improves symptoms. Some women find relief by taking a vitamin E supplement (400 International Units) twice daily.

Hormonal Headaches

Estrogen may trigger headaches and migraines among some women, particularly those with a history of migraines. Reducing the dose of estrogen often relieves the headaches. In one study of eighty-seven women who experienced migraine headaches while receiving estrogen, 58 percent experienced a reduction in symptoms after the dosage of estrogen was reduced. Taking a nonoral type of androgen along with estrogen often helps, too.

Sensitivity to Estrogen

Although rare, some women are allergic to estrogen, developing such unusual symptoms as hyperactivity or even severe abdominal pain. If your doctor suspects you have a sensitivity to estrogen, he or she may recommend that you try a different type of estrogen or a different route of administration. If these changes fail to solve the problem, you may be advised to stop taking estrogen altogether.

CHAPTER 11

❧

Do You Really Need Hormone Therapy?

Since estrogen additive therapy (and probably combined estrogen-progestogen therapy) can ease your menopausal symptoms, improve your odds against developing heart disease, and protect against osteoporosis, why shouldn't *all* women take postmenopausal hormone therapy? Frankly because taking estrogen is not the only way to relieve the discomforts of menopause and to prevent heart disease and osteoporosis. Diet and exercise provide ample protection against heart disease, and a lifetime of exercise and good eating habits protects against osteoporosis as well.

If you can't take postmenopausal estrogens—or don't want or need to take them—there are plenty of things you can do to make your middle years more comfortable and to keep healthy in your later years, as we have pointed out throughout this book. Even if you *do* take hormones, we believe hormone therapy should be considered an *adjunct* to such life-style habits as a low-fat diet that's adequate in calcium, and regular exercise, not a substitute for them.

Whatever you decide, make sure you are regularly monitored by your physician. If you decide not to take hormone therapy, your physician will want to ensure that an indication (such as accelerated bone loss) doesn't develop later on. If you do decide to take hormone therapy, you should be monitored to ensure that the treatment is effective, safe, and not producing any serious side effects. Keep in mind, too, that it's never too late to start taking estrogen. So even if you decide *not* to take it now, you can always change your mind later on.

Estrogen: yes or no? The choice is up to you. Now that you have the facts and the information you need, you can (with the help of your doctor) make an informed, intelligent decision.

Appendix

Menopausal Symptoms Questionnaire

Grading System: Please Assess Symptoms Listed Below According to the Following Symbols:

A = No symptoms

B = Mild; symptoms experienced, but not severe enough to warrant treatment

C = Moderate; symptoms make you feel uncomfortable to the extent that you would like treatment

D = Severe; symptoms interfere with your daily living style; you feel you *need* treatment.

Symptoms

Hot flashes_____

   How many/day?_____

   How many/week?_____

Perspiration_____

Palpitations_____

Insomnia:

   Difficulty getting

     to sleep_____

   Early awakening_____

Mood change_____

Irritability_____

Depression_____

Vaginal itching_____

   Burning_____

Vaginal discharge_____

   Dryness_____

Intercourse:

   Painful_____

   Difficult_____

   Frequency/week_____

     Increased_____

     Decreased_____

Interest in sex:

   Same_____

   Increased_____

   Decreased_____

Other Symptoms

_____

_____

_____

_____

Factors That Aggravate or Improve Symptoms

1. Are the above symptoms made worse by stress?

Yes___No___

If yes, type of stress:_____

2. Are the above symptoms made worse by any other events?

Yes___No___

If yes, briefly note:_____

3. Are you on, or have you recently been on hormones or other treatment? Yes___No___

4. Did your symptoms improve/worsen on treatment?
Symptoms: Increased___Decreased___Same___

5. Symptoms that were improved/worsened. Use same grading as before.

Symptom Grade Before Treatment While on Treatment

_____

_____

6. Remarks regarding symptoms not mentioned above:

_____
_____
_____
_____
_____
_____
_____

Calcium Questionnaire

For each of the following foods you consumed in the last three days, estimate the total amount for each day and write it in columns 1, 2, and 3 (e.g., ½ cup, 6 oz., 5 tbsp., etc.). Then calculate your total calcium intake for the three days by multiplying the amount of calcium in a single serving by the number of servings you had. Add up the total amount of calcium you ate, then divide that number by three. This will give you an estimate of your daily calcium intake. Compare your daily intake with the recommended intakes for women below.

Dairy Products

	Serving Size	Calcium (mg)	1	2	3	Total
MILK Whole	1 c.	288				
Low fat (2%)	1 c.	352				
Skim & Buttermilk	1 c.	296				
Nonfat, dry	¼ c.	220				
Chocolate	1 c.	278				
Condensed, sweetened	1 c.	802				
Evaporated	1 c.	635				
Lactimilk	1 c.	300				

	Serving Size	Calcium (mg)	1	2	3	Total
CHEESE						
Swiss	1 oz.	262				
Cheddar, Provolone	1 oz.	213				
Edam	1 oz.	207				
Monterey Jack, Mozzarella	1 oz.	200				
Muenster	1 oz.	200				
American, Gouda	1 oz.	198				
Brick	1 oz.	191				
Velveeta (cheese food) 2 tbsp.=	1 oz.	162				
Romano	1 oz.	156				
Blue	1 oz.	150				
Parmesan	1 oz.	136				
Feta	1 oz.	100				
Ricotta (skim)	1 oz.	84				
Ricotta (whole)	1 oz.	65				
Brie	1 oz.	52				
Camembert	1 oz.	30				
Cottage, low fat	1 c.	204				
Cottage, regular	1 c.	131				
OTHER						
Ice cream (hard)	1 c.	194				
Ice cream (soft)	1 c.	253				
Ice milk (hard)	1 c.	204				

	Serving Size	Calcium (mg)	1	2	3	Total
Pudding (instant)	1 c.	374				
Pudding (cooked)	1 c.	265				
Custard (baked)	1 c.	297				
Yogurt, low fat plain	1 c.	452				
Yogurt, low fat fruited	1 c.	313				
Yogurt, whole milk	1 c.	275				
Yogurt, frozen	1 c.	220				

Seafood

	Serving Size	Calcium (mg)	1	2	3	Total
Clams, canned (solid/liquid)	1 c.	121				
Mackerel, canned (solid/liquid)	1 c.	552				
Oyster stew (milk, 6 oysters)	1 c.	274				
Salmon, sockeye, canned (solid, liquid w/bones)	1 c.	587				
Sardines, canned (w/bones)	4 med.	69				

Vegetables & Nuts

	Serving Size	Calcium (mg)	1	2	3	Total
Broccoli (frozen, chopped, cooked)	1 c.	100				
Bok choy (chopped, cooked)	1 c.	250				
Collards (frozen, chopped, cooked)	1 c.	299				
Kale (frozen, chopped, cooked)	1 c.	157				
Mustard greens (frozen, chopped, cooked)	1 c.	156				
Turnip greens (frozen, chopped, cooked)	1 c.	195				
Beans, all types (dry, cooked, canned, solid/ liquid)	1 c.	80				
Almonds (shelled, chopped)	1 c.	304				
Pecans (shelled, chopped)	1 c.	86				
Peanuts (shelled)	1 c.	104				
Mixed nuts, dry roasted peanuts	1 c.	96				
Walnuts, English (shelled, chopped)	1 c.	119				

Miscellaneous

	Serving Size	Calcium (mg)	1	2	3	Total
Tofu	1 oz.	36				
Soybeans (cooked, sprouted)	1 c.	54				
Sunflower seeds (hulled)	1 c.	174				
Cream soups (made with milk)	1 c.	184				
Macaroni & cheese (home-made)	1 c.	362				
Pizza (frozen w/cheese)	4.5″ arc	89				
Carob flour	1 c.	480				
Molasses, black-strap	1 tbsp.	137				

Calcium-Fortified Foods

	Serving Size	Calcium (mg)	1	2	3	Total
Minute Maid orange juice	1 c.	320				
Calci-Milk	1 c.	500				

Total Calcium   ———

Average Daily Calcium Intake   ———
(Divide Total Calcium by 3)

Recommended Calcium Intake for Women

Age	Recommended Daily Intake (mg)
Children (age 1-10)	800
Adolescents (age 11-18)	1,200
Pregnant/lactating women over age 20	1,200
Premenopause (to age 35 with functioning ovaries)	800-1,000
Perimenopause (age 35-50 with functioning ovaries)	1,000-1,200
Postmenopausal (natural or surgical menopause)	1,400-2,000

How to Examine Your Breasts

When examining your breasts, you may notice that your breast tissue naturally feels lumpy. You may be wondering how to differentiate between "normal" lumpiness and a lump you should report to your doctor. Once you've made BSE a regular habit, you'll be better able to tell the difference between what's normal and what's not. One way to keep track is to record "troublesome" areas on a diagram, much like your physician does. We've provided a diagram here for you to use (Figure A-1). As you examine your breasts, make a note of any areas that feel "soft," "firm," "thick," or "grainy" (or choose another term that best describes what you feel). The next time you examine your breasts, you can refer back to the diagram and compare what you feel with your previous BSE.

FIGURE A-1. Breast Diagram for Keeping Track of What You Feel During BSE

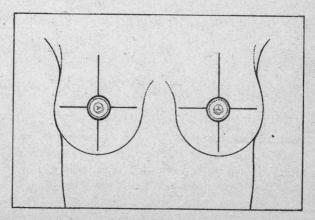

Visual Examination

Stand in front of the mirror and look at your breasts. They should be about the same size and shape. (Many women have one breast that is slightly larger than the other.)

Place your hands on your hips and push down. Do you notice any changes? A pulling in one area? Next, lean over slightly and continue to look for any differences in the two breasts.

Now raise your hands above your head and press your palms together. Again, look to see if there is any difference between the two breasts. Look for dimpling of the skin, abnormal bulges or pulling, areas of redness, or what is called "orange peel" skin. Look at the nipple. Does it pull inward? If you see any of these abnormal signs, make a note of it on your diagram and have your breasts checked by your physician.

FIGURE A-2. Starting Position for BSE

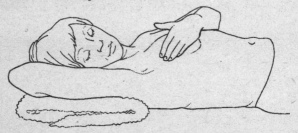

Manual Examination

Lie down and place a small pillow or folded towel behind your back on the right side. Raise your right arm over your head or place your right hand behind your head (Figure A-2). Using one of the BSE patterns illustrated here

(Figure A-3), examine your right breast with your left hand. Use the flat part of your fingers to examine your breast (Figure A-4), *not* your fingertips (Figure A-5). Now, moving your fingers in a circular motion, feel the breast tissue lightly, then more deeply. Be sure to feel the upper chest areas; the area just under the breast, and the area under your arms just as carefully as you examine the breast itself. When you have completed the examination on one side, repeat the procedure on the other, remembering to move the pillow or towel to the other side. Now repeat the examination sitting upright. You are looking and feeling for lumps that are not normal. Remember, every woman's breasts have some areas that may feel thickened or grainy. This is especially true as you grow older. A lump that is not normal may be any size. It may move around freely or be fixed. If you find something unusual, see your physician.

FIGURE A-3. Patterns to follow during BSE
A

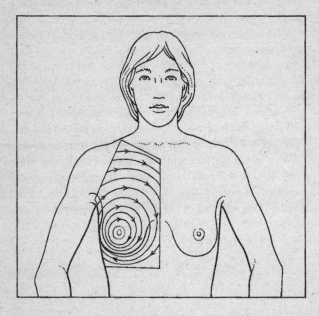

B

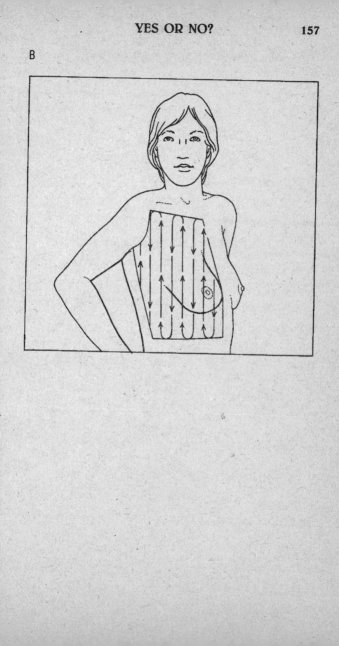

FIGURE A-4. Correct Placement of Fingers for BSE

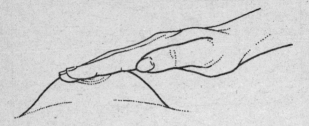

FIGURE A-5. Incorrect Placement of Fingers for BSE

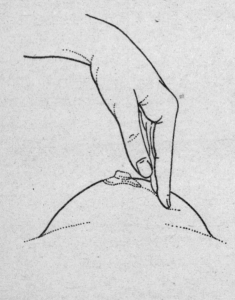

Postmenopausal Hormone Preparations

Oral Estrogens

Brand Name	Type of Estrogen	Available Dosages	Manufacturer
Premarin	Conjugated equine estrogens	0.3 mg 0.625 mg 0.9 mg 1.25 mg 2.5 mg	Ayerst
Estrace	Micronized estradiol	1.0 mg 2.0 mg	Mead Johnson
Estratab	Esterified estrogens	0.3 mg 0.625 mg 1.25 mg 2.5 mg	Solvay
Ogen	Estropipate	0.625 mg 1.25 mg 2.5 mg 5.0 mg	Abbott
Estinyl	Ethinyl estradiol	0.02 mg 0.05 mg 0.5 mg	Schering
Estrovis	Quinestrol	0.1 mg	Parke-Davis

Estrogen Vaginal Creams

Premarin	Conjugated equine estrogens	0.625 mg	Ayerst
Estrace	17beta-estradiol	0.1 mg	Mead Johnson
Ogen	Estropipate	1.5 mg	Abbott
Ortho Dienestrol	Dienestrol	0.01%	Ortho

| Estragard | Dienestrol | 0.01% | Solvay |
| Diethyl stilbestrol suppositories | Diethylstilbestrol | 0.1mg 0.5mg | Lilly |

Parenteral Estrogens (Injections, Pellets, Patches)

Depo-Estradiol	Estradiol cypionate	1 mg	Upjohn
Delestrogen	Estradiol valerate	10 mg 20 mg 40 mg	Squibb
Estraval	Estradiol valerate	10 mg 20 mg	Solvay
Estrapel	Estradiol pellet	25 mg pellet	Bartor
Estraderm	Transdermal estradiol	0.05 mg/ day 0.1 mg/ day	Ciba-Geigy

Progestogens

Provera	Medroxyprogesterone acetate	10 mg	Upjohn
Curretab	Medroxyprogesterone acetate	10 mg	Solvay
Cyrin	Medroxyprogesterone acetate	10 mg	Ayerst
Amen	Medroxyprogesterone acetate	10 mg	Carnick
Aygestin	Norethindrone acetate	5 mg	Ayerst
Norlutate	Norethindrone acetate	5 mg	Parke-Davis

Norlutin	Norethindrone	5 mg	Parke-Davis
Megace	Megesterol acetate	20 mg 40 mg	Bristol-Myers
Ovrette	Norgestrel	0.075 mg	Wyeth
Micronor	Norethindrone	0.35 mg	Ortho
Nor-Q.D.	Norethindrone	0.35 mg	Syntex
	Micronized oral progesterone	100 mg	
	Progesterone vaginal suppositories	25 mg 50 mg	

Oral Androgens

Oreton	Methyltestosterone	5 mg	Schering
Metandren	Methyltestosterone	5 mg	Ciba
Halotestin	Fluoxymesterone	5 mg	Upjohn
Fluoxy-mesterone	Fluoxymesterone	5 mg	Solvay
Ora-Testryl	Fluoxymesterone	5 mg	Squibb

Injectable Androgens

Depo-testosterone	Testosterone cypionate	50 mg/ml	Upjohn
Depo-testadiol			
Delatestryl	Testosterone enanthate	100 mg/ml	Squibb

Androgen Pellets

| Testopel | Testosterone pellets | 75 mg | Bartor |

Androgen Ointments

	Testosterone propionate	2% in a petrolatum base	

Estrogen Androgen Combinations

Estratest tablets	Esterified estrogens	1.25 mg	Solvay
	Methyltestosterone	2.5 mg	
Estratest H.S. tablets	Esterified estrogens	0.625 mg	Solvay
	Methyltestosterone	1.25 mg	
Premarin with Methyl-testosterone	Conjugated equine estrogens	1.25 mg	Ayerst
	Methyltestosterone	10 mg	
Premarin with methyl-testosterone	Conjugated equine estrogens	0.625 mg	Ayerst
	Methyltestosterone	5 mg	
Depo-Testadiol	Estradiol cypionate	2 mg	Upjohn
	Testosterone cypionate	50 mg	

Tables adapted with permission from Gambrell, R.D., *Estrogen Replacement Therapy.* Essential Medical Systems, Inc. 1990.

INDEX

✿

Page numbers of illustrations and tables appear in italics

About the Authors

MORRIS NOTELOVITZ, M.D., Ph.D., was the founder of the Center for Climacteric Studies, based at the University of Florida at Gainesville. In 1986 he opened the Women's Medical and Diagnostic Center and Climacteric Clinic to provide medical care for pre- and postmenopausal women. Since 1980, Dr. Notelovitz has supervised research and clinical management on more than 11,000 women age thirty and over, focusing on issues of menopause. He is the author of *Stand Tall: An Informed Woman's Guide to Preventing Osteoporosis.*

DIANA TONNESSEN is a free-lance writer on health and science issues. Her work has appeared in *Health*, *McCalls*, and elsewhere. She is the coauthor with Dr. Morris Notelovitz of *Menopause and Midlife Health.*